ADDRESSES AND ESSAYS ON VEGETARIANISM

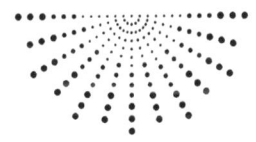

ANNA BONUS KINGSFORD

CONTENTS

1. SOCIAL CONSIDERATIONS — 1
2. LETTERS ON PURE DIET — 7
3. A LECTURE ON FOOD — 29
4. THE BEST FOOD FOR MAN — 71
5. THE PHYSIOLOGY OF VEGETARIANISM — 92
6. HISTORICAL ASPECT OF FOOD REFORM — 102
7. SOME ASPECTS OF THE VEGETARIAN QUESTION — 110
8. FROM ADDRESSES TO VEGETARIANS — 146
9. EVOLUTION AND FLESH-EATING — 157

O CONSIDER THIS, YE THAT EAT FLESH.

"The Lord will abhor both the bloodthirsty and deceitful man. (...) Their inward parts are very wickedness. Their throat is an open sepulchre."

— (*PSALMS* 5:7-10)

"They are corrupt, they have done abominable works, there is none that doeth good. The LORD looked down from heaven upon the children of men, to see if there were any that did understand, and seek God. They are all gone out of the way, they are altogether become filthy".

— (*PSALMS* 14:1-3).

"Their throat is an open sepulcher. (...) Their feet are swift to shed blood. Destruction and unhappiness are in their ways, and the way of peace have they not known. There is no fear of God before their eyes."

— (*ROMANS* 3:15-18)

"I will take no bullock out of thy house: nor he goats out of thy folds. For every beast of the forest is mine, and so are the cattle upon a thousand hills. I know all the fouls of the mountains: and the wild beasts of the field are mine. If I were hungry, I would not tell thee: for the whole world is mine, and all that is therein. Will I eat the flesh of bulls, or drink the blood of goats?"

— (*PSALMS* 50:9-13)

"What dost thou preach my laws, and takest my covenant in thy mouth? Seeing thou hatest instruction, and casteth my words behind thee. (…) thou thoughtest wickedly, that I am even such a one as thyself (…) Now consider this, ye that forget God".

— (*PSALMS* 50:16-22)

"AS FOR ME, I WILL WALK INNOCENTLY."

— (*PSALMS* 26:11)

1. SOCIAL CONSIDERATIONS

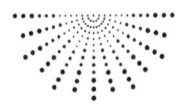

Is[1] it morally lawful for cultivated and refined persons to impose upon a whole class of the population a disgusting, brutalising, and unwholesome occupation, which is scientifically and experimentally demonstrable to be not merely entirely needless, but absolutely inimical to the best interests of the human race?

Butchers are the Pariahs of the western world; the very name itself of their trade has become a synonym for barbarity, and is used as a term of reproach in speaking of persons notorious for brutality, coarseness, of love of bloodshed. The common exclamation, "What a butcher is So-and-so!" in reference to such men, betrays the horror and reprobation with which are instinctively regarded the followers of a trade created and patronized chiefly by the "refined" classes!

In the report of a "diseased meat" case given in the **Leeds Mercury** of 6th March 1880, the ensuing passage occurs: –

"Mr. J. Ellis, President of the Leeds Butchers' Association, stated that there was no disease about the lungs of the animal at all. Blood had probably been forced into them by some person jumping on the animal's body after it had been felled.

"Mr. Bruce: Is it a common practice ***when a beast in dying*** for a person to jump upon it to force the blood out of it?

"Witness: Yes."

In the course of the celebrated Tichborne case a certain metropolitan butcher was called to testify to the claimant's identity. This man averred that *employés* in slaughter-houses habitually make use of clogs to avoid soaking their feet in the pools of blood which continually inundate the pavements of these places. Really, when one thinks of these unfortunate and brutalised men, thus condemned by modern "civilisation" – Heaven save the mark! – to pass their days in the midst of spectacles and practices so foul and loathsome, taking part daily in wholesome massacres, and living only to take away life, it is impossible not to conclude that such men are deprived of all chance of becoming themselves civilised, and are consequently disinherited of their human rights and defrauded of their human dignity. And not only the slaughterers themselves, but all those who are directly of indirectly associated with this abominable traffic – cattle-drivers and dealers, meat-salesmen, their apprentices and clerks – all these live in familiar, if not exclusive, contact with practices and sights of the vilest and most hideous kind; all these are condemned to the degradation or suppression of the most characteristic features of Humanity.

With people in general, the very look and touch of raw flesh excite a disgust which only a special education can overcome. So that in the butchers and cook persons are condemned to work which their employers deem altogether repulsive. It is absurd to suppose that if kreophagy were really natural to mankind, the sentiment in regard to butchers and their trade, to which allusion has been made, would find such spontaneous and universal expression among us. The true carnivora and omnivora have no horror of dead bodies; the sight of blood, the smell of raw flesh, inspires them with no manner of disgust. If all of us, men and women alike, were compelled to dispense with the offices of a paid slaughterer an to immolate our victims with our own hands, the ***penchant*** for flesh would not long survive in polite society. It would be indeed hard to find a man or woman of the upper or middle classes who would willingly consent to undertake the butcher's duties, and go the cattle-yard armed with pole-axe or knife to fell an ox or to slit the throat of a sheep or lamb, or even of a rabbit, for the morrow's repast. On the other hand, there is no one, however delicately bred or refined, who would not readily take a basket and gather apples in an orchard or peaches in a garden, or who, if need should arise, would object to make a cake or an omelette.

It would, alas! require many long pages to cite the innumerable cruelties and sufferings which the gluttony and luxury of flesh-eating man impose on the innocent herb-feeders – sufferings which, whatever may be said to the contrary, are ***absolutely inevitable*** and inseparable from modern European habits of diet. Sufferings by sea and land, in transit from different ports, by rail and by road, sufferings in the live-stock markets, in the pens of the slaughter-houses while waiting their turn for death, sufferings by thirst, blows, terror, apprehension, exhaustion, neglect, to say nothing of the wanton barbarity to which they are too often subjected, such, under the present hateful and unnatural system, is the woeful lot of the patient, gentle, laborious creatures who should be ploughing our fields, and yielding us, not their flesh and blood, but milk and wool and the fruits of their willing toil. [2]

1. From ***The Prefect Way in Diet***, by Anna Kingsford (New Edition, 1897, pp. 61-64). See *Biographical Preface*, p. 42, *ante*.
2. Here follow harrowing details, given by various ewe-witnesses, of cruelties and sufferings connected with and inseparable from the cattle-traffic and the slaughter-house.

An Act consolidating and amending the law as to cruelty to animals has recently been passed. By section I of the Protection of Animals Act 1911, provision is made for the punishment of persons who shall be convicted of certain acts of cruelty, therein specified, to domestic or captive animals, as therein defined, but the same section contains a proviso in favour of (*inter alia*) "***the destruction, or preparation for destruction, of any animal as food for mankind***": and in favour of coursing and hunting captive animals, and in favour of legalized vivisection. The effect of this Act is to enlarge the class of legally protected animals, but, unless a more liberal and humane construction is put upon it than was put upon the former Act – the Prevention of Cruelty to Animals Act 1849 – which also was passed with the object of protecting certain animals against cruelty and ill-treatment, it will be but a poor protection: for, the judges, having decided that the former Act was direct against only **unnecessary abuse**, that is, abuse which flesh-eaters would consider to be unnecessary – held, that an act such as the branding of the lambs on nose with a hot iron for the purpose of their identification, was not cruel: and, while the very painful operation of dishorning cattle by sawing off their horns close to their heads for the purpose of slightly increasing their value, and for convenience in feeding and packing, was held by an English judge to be unnecessary and cruel, and therefore unjustifiable; judges in Scotland and Ireland declined to follow such holding, and decided that dishorning cattle was not an offence! It was urged, on behalf of the practice of dishorning cattle, that it made them graze better and fatten more quickly. When, in the first instance, this case came before the justices, they found that the farmer who had dishorned the cattle had "acted under the belief that the operation ***was for the benefit of the animals themselves*** as well as for his own benefit as grazer." It was held, under the old Act, that a painful operation performed on an animal, ***benefiting the owner by increasing the values of the animal***, was not legally cruel, even though the operation was in fact unnecessary and useless (e.g. the operation of spaying sows). Such was the construction put by flesh-eating judges on an Act passed for the Prevention of Cruelty to Animals! It will be observed that all these cruelties were done for and on behalf of the flesh-eaters as such. For how long is this state of things to continue? So degraded has this nation of England become under a regime of flesh, that such wantonly cruel and heartless acts as the following can be openly perpetrated without remonstrance of fear of punishment, and without adverse comment in a daily paper giving publicity to them. The **Daily Express**, of 2nd November 1911, without a word of condemnation or disapprobation, says: "A seal was seen in the Thames yesterday [All Saints Day] and chased into the Higham Canal, which joins the river at Gravesend. It was pelted with stones and finally shot." – S.H.H.

2. LETTERS ON PURE DIET

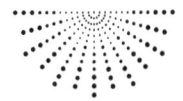

I

IT[1] is with the most earnest satisfaction, and presage of good things to come, that all Food Reformers scattered over the United Kingdom will welcome this first appearance of a Metropolitan Journal devoted to the propagation of our faith and practice. The system we advocate is pre-eminently a scientific system, and for that very reason, it requires special organisation and special exposition to make known its bases and its value. The poor are too ignorant to comprehend its **rationale**, the rich are too indolent or too luxurious to care to trouble themselves about the subject; it is chiefly among the middle class that our teaching is likely to find minds capable of understanding and hearts of being touched. For our system, whether we call it Dietetic Reform, Vegetarianism, or Pythagoreanism, is not **all** scientific. It appeals to the intuitional as well as to the intellectual faculties; and it is hard to say in which direction the appeal is stronger.

On the one hand we are able to command the advocacy of Comparative Anatomy and Physiology, Chemistry, Hygiene, and Economy Social and Political; on the other, our cause is pleaded by all the arts which beautify life and civilise humanity, and – better and worthier still than these – by those just, compassionate, and gentle instincts of man, in virtue of which alone he *is* man, differing from and surpassing all lower creatures.

The Perfectionist is necessarily an abstainer from flesh. No man who aims at making his life an harmonious whole, pure, complete, and harmless to others, can endure to gratify an appetite at the cost of the daily suffering and bloodshed of his inferiors in degree, and of the moral degradation of his own kind. I know not which strikes me most forcibly in the ethics of this question –the ***injustice***, the ***cruelty***, or the ***nastiness*** of flesh-eating. The injustice is to the butchers, the cruelty is to the animals, the nastiness concerns the consumer. With regard to this last in particular, I greatly wonder that persons of refinement – aye, even of decency – do not feel insulted on being offered, as a matter of course, portions of corpses as food! Such comestibles might possibly be tolerated during sieges, or times of other privation of proper viands in exceptional circumstances, but in the midst of a civilised community able to command a profusion of sound and delicious foods, it ought to be deemed an affront to set dead flesh before a guest.

What disfigurement, too, this horrible practice of corpse-eating causes in otherwise civilised cities, replete with beautiful monuments, cathedrals, fountains, avenues, and all kinds of decorative art; where, side by with pictures, flowers, jewels, statues and embroideries, one meets at intervals of every few yards the loathsome, foul, and indecent spectacle of slaughtered bullocks, sheep, pigs, and other animals hanging in rows, exposed to public view, the blood often trickling down from their mutilated trunks, and coagulating on the pavement!

To me it is simply amazing that human society should tolerate these things, and still more amazing that the person who objects to put carrion into this mouth should be seriously expected to adopt the position of an apologist, and required to make good his case! Surely the case makes itself sufficiently "good" on the face of it; and assuredly, also, the burden of excuse lies, not with the pure food-eater, but with the eater of flesh. **He** it is who is the innovator, **he** it is who has departed from the law of nature and from the customs of his ancestors! Shew me then, O man of prey, for what reason you slit the throat of a living creature and devour its tissues and organs, when you may have nourishment of better value, in purer and stronger condition, without recourse to bloodshed! Shew me why you are not revolted and shocked by the contemplation of all the filthy practices and processes involved in this habit of carnage; how you reconcile the idea of the slaughter-house with ideas of progress, beauty, and gentle manners; and when you have made out your case to your satisfaction, it will be time enough for me to begin making out mine!

We all know the story of the butcher who coaxed his little son to repeat the Church Catechism on Sunday by promising that if he said it nicely he should be allowed to kill a lamb before breakfast on Monday morning. Everybody, on hearing this story, express horror and disgust at the notion of so dreadful a bribe being held out to a child in reward for the performance of a religious exercise. But why? In reason's name, why? If the slaughter of lambs be a virtuous and humanising business, why should not the child be initiated into his father's craft as early and as innocently as into any other? If the boy had been promised the treat of baking a loaf or planing a piece of wood by way of reward for his good conduct, the story would have shocked nobody. But, admit that slaughtering is a horrible business in itself, and the instinctive disgust becomes at once explicable. That which is base for the man is, of course, doubly vile for the innocent child.

As I write, I chance to light on a passage from a modern romance, and cannot forbear quoting from it, with slight alteration, a few portions, so well it puts one aspect of the moral side of our question.

"Cookery the divine, can turn a horrible fact into a poetic idealism, can twine the butcher's knife with lilies, and hide a carcase under roses. Men write stanzas of 'gush' on 'maternity,' and tear the little bleating calf from its mother to bleed to death in a long slow agony; send the spring-tide lamb to the slaughter; have scores of birds and beasts slain for one dinner, that they may enjoy the numberless dishes which fashion exacts; and then – all the time talking softly about *rissôle* and *mayonnaise*, *consommé* and *entremet*, *croquette* and *côtelette*, the dear gourmets thank God that they are not as the parded beasts of prey! (...) If there be a spectacle on earth to rejoice the angels, it is not man's treatment of the animals he says God has given to him! I wonder if ever He ask how men have dealt with His gift, what they will answer! If all their slaughtered millions should answer instead of them, if all the countless and unpitied dead, all the goaded, maddened beasts from forest and desert, and all the innocent, playful little home-bred creatures that have been racked by the knives and torn by the poisons and convulsed by the torments of modern science, should answer instead – what then? If, with one mighty voice of a woe no longer inarticulate, of an accusation no longer disregarded, these oxen with their blood-shot, agonised eyes, driven to death in the slaughter-house; these sheep with their timid, woe-begone faces, scourged into the place of their doom, bruised, terrified, and tortured, should answer instead – what then? Then, if it be done unto men as they have done unto these, they will seek for mercy and find none in all the width of the universe, they will moan and none shall release, they will pray, and none shall hear."

Well, two classes of men are chiefly to blame for all this demoralisation and suffering: the clergy, and the physicians. Both have erred and continue to err for lack of education and discernment on the one hand; and on the other, for sake of the love of popularity and power. But these questions are deep ones, and will involve a more careful and particular study than, in the limits of the present article, I am able to give them. They will form good subjects for examination at a future time, when I trust to be able to speak at some length of the true bearing both of sacred scripture and of therapeutic science on the question of flesh-eating, and to make it clear that the misapprehension which exists so widely with regard to the teaching of these two authorities, is due, not to the authorities themselves, but to misconception and misinterpretation on the part of their expositors.

II

We may assume that the public interested in the Food Question – as in every other national question – is divisible into three sections, namely, the section led by ecclesiastical opinion, that led by medical opinion, and lastly, the independent or free thinking section which either despises or ignores the opinions of both clergy and "doctors."

It may seem at first sight a strange thing that the advocate of pure diet should have any difficulties to contend with on religious grounds; but those who are experienced in the campaign of Food Reform, know well that the average Christian, of whatever denomination, commonly regards the doctrine of abstinence from flesh as an arrant heresy. He quotes Paul on the subject, hurls Peter's vision at ones head, and triumphantly cites what he assumes to have been the practice of the Founder himself of Christianity, evidence, which for him, would clinch the argument, even if Moses and the Hebrew code of clean and unclean beasts had never been heard of. What, in the face of such arguments, is to be the reply of our advocate?

Let us deal first with the head and front of the

difficulty; its minor points may be set in order afterwards.

Most modern Christians believe that Jesus ate not only fish, but flesh, and this impression constitutes for them clear licence and sanction to do likewise, although a careful examination of the Sacred Writings and a scrupulous comparison of the various statements made in the Gospels would go far to convince them that the probabilities of the case are strongly in favour of a wholly different view.

In the second chapter of Matthew it is stated that Jesus was a "Nazarene." The fact that the writer refers to prophecy for his authority plainly shows that he means not a Nazarene in the sense of a mere inhabitant of Nazareth, but a "Nazarite," for the reference made can only be to the declaration of Jacob (**Genesis**, chap. Xlix, verse 26), in which the word **nâzîr** occurs for the first time in the Bible, and in the Protestant version is translated **"separate"**; to the directions given by an angel to the mother of Samson; and to the vow of Hannah in regard to Samuel. According to ecclesiastical tradition, a Nazarene, or Nazarite, appears to have been one who wore his hair long, clothed himself in a single outer garment without seam, abstained from fermented drinks,[2] and, in the higher degrees of the order, as among the Essenes, from flesh-meats also, after the manner of John the Baptist. The belief that

Jesus was one of this order is not only supported by Gospel statement, but by legendary art, based on early conviction and doctrine, as is conclusively shewn by all the Christian representations of the Master, depicting Him invariably in the Nazarite garb, with flowing hair and beard. That He was an adherent of John's doctrine appears further probable from the fact that He sought and underwent baptism at the hands of the latter, and the very word "**Essene**" is derived from a root signifying "**Bather**." To be "**bathed**" was, therefore, to profess Essenism.

There is no evidence, written or traditional, that Jesus ever partook of flesh. The phrase, "the Son of Man is come eating and drinking," is plainly shewn by the context (in the revised edition) to refer to the eating of **bread**; and it implies that Jesus did not push abstinence to asceticism, as did John. The Paschal Lamb difficulty (in connection with the Last Supper) arises out of a simple misunderstanding, easily rectifiable. The Last Supper is shown in the gospel of John, who himself was a prominent figure on the occasion,[3] to have taken place on the evening of the thirteenth day of the month of Nisan, that is, as is many times distinctly affirmed, **before** the day of the Paschal meal, which was the fourteenth of Nisan. On this latter day (Friday) the Crucifixion itself took place, for we are told in all four Gospels that this event occurred on the preparation day of the Sabbath, which Sabbath, being also the Convocation day, was "an high day." The date of the Crucifixion is unmistakably fixed by John in the verse: "They led Jesus, therefore, into the palace (or pretorium); and it was early; and they themselves entered not into the palace, that they might not be defiled, **but might eat the Passover**." That the Crucifixion took place the day after that of the Last Supper is clearly stated by all four Evangelists, and this fact affords plain evidence that the mention of the "eating of the Passover" in relation to the Supper is an erroneous interpolation, for all of them agree that it was held on the thirteenth of Nisan (Thursday), on which day the Passover **could not have been eaten**.

But that Jesus ate fish is, if the Gospel records are to be accepted in their literal sense – **an assumption I emphatically contest** – pretty well established. Let me point out the strong indications which exist why the fish-eating and fish-catching attributed to Jesus and His disciples have, not a literal, but a parabolic and mystic meaning, precisely as have also the many references to the "cup" and to wine-drinking in the same narratives. All these allusions are related to astronomical symbology, and identify the Hero of the Christian Evangels with His ancient prototypes. It is admitted by most critics of the Sacred Scriptures that they are largely base on and governed by reference to that science, which, in earlier times, and in Eastern lands – whence both the Hebrew and Christian oracles are derived – dominated and directed all expressions, whether tabular or written of psychic truths. The science was founded on the study of the Celestial Planisphere, and its earliest and most universal text-book was the Zodiac. The phenomenon known as the Precession of the Equinoxes causes a different sign in the Zodiac to appear at the vernal equinox about every two thousand years, and to the character of this vernal sign, prominent expression was given by the initiated, in the theological cultus of the period. Thus history has shewn us successively the Bull (Apis) and the Lamb (Aries) as the dominant emblems of Egyptian and Jewish worship; and this latter sign has survived in Christian symbolism because Aries is always the first Zodiacal hieroglyph, and thus the permanent emblem of the one eternal year or great Sun-cycle. But the sign which actually ushered in the Christian dispensation, and which, therefore, we should expect to find reflected in the sacred legends of the period, was **Pisces**, or the Fish. Hence the Messiah, who appeared under the auspices of this sign, is portrayed as being followed by Fishers; as distributing Fishes ("the two small fishes" of the Zodiac) to His disciples; as preparing Fish for the food of His Apostles; and as Himself partaking of Fish after His resurrection. Besides, the fish is the maritime emblem, and Jesus is said to have been born of

Maria and the Holy Ghost, or of Water and the Spirit. The prophet Esdras (**Esdras**, book ii, chap. 13) sees Christ in a vision coming up out of the sea; and the ceremony of "passing through the sea and the cloud" is still connected with the initiation into Christian doctrine. For these reasons, the Kingdom of Heaven is likened to a Net, and the Apostles are told they should be "fishers of men." Clement of Alexandria writes to his people early in the third century: "Let our signets be a Dove (the Holy Spirit), or a Fish (symbol of the water), or the heavenward-sailing Ship, or the Lyre (of the Sea-nymph), or the Anchor." All these symbols are found in the Celestial Planisphere. In the Roman catacombs – the home of primitive Christian art – the most remarkable and the most general symbol employed to express the name of Christ was that of the Fish, which affords, significatively, a combination of everything desirable in a tessera, or mystic sign. The Greek word for fish – **'ΙΧΘΥΣ** – contains the initials of the words – **'Ιησους ΧρισΤὸς θεοῦ Ὑιος ΣωΤήρ** (Jesus Christ, Son of God, the Saviour). Sometimes the word **'Ιχθυς** was written at length in place of the graven symbol. Augustine also applies this emblem to Jesus, and says that "He is a Fish which lives in the midst of waters." Paulinus, speaking of the miracle of the five loaves and two fishes (the mystic number of planets), alludes to Jesus as "the Fish of the Living waters." Prosper refers to Him as "the Fish dressed at his death." And Tertullian calls the Christians "fishes bred in the water, and saved by one great Fish." Jerome, commending a disciple who sought baptism, tells him that, "like the Son of the Fish, he desires to be cast into the water." As thus the Messiah of the Gospels is associated with the sea and with redemption through and by water, so, with perfect reason, the successors of Peter, His chief apostle and vicar, claim as their distinctive title the name of the "Fisherman," and the ring with which each successive Pontiff is invested, in token of his office and authority, is known as the "Fisherman's Ring." It has been observed also that the mitre, characteristic of ecclesiastical authority in the Christian Church, represents a fish's head, and expresses, therefore, the relation of the wearer to the Founder of the religion inaugurated under that sign. Fish were connected in primitive Christian times with all theological ceremonies; the Saints in the sacred mysteries were called **"*pisciculi*"** (little fishes), and to this day the water vase at the entrance of Catholic Churches bears the name of **"*piscina.*"** The custom of eating fish on Friday, in commemoration of the chief event in the history of Him whose Mother is identical with the genius of that day, is still common in the larger section of Christians.

We might insist at greater length on the peculiarly symbolical character of the whole twenty-first chapter of John's Gospel containing the account of the final fish-miracle, which chapter is appended as an epilogue to the Gospel itself, whose formally concluding verse closes the preceding chapter. More than one critic has pointed out the strong probability that the episode referred to, with its curiously emphasised numerals, – seven, two hundred, a hundred and fifty and three – and the unlikely character of its literal interpretation (see the Rev. Malcolm White on the symbolical numbers of Scripture), is altogether mystical and, perhaps, prophetical in meaning. But enough has been said to indicate the reasons for attaching a sense, not historical but symbolical, to the various statements contained in the four Gospels on the subject of Christ's connection with fish and fishery, and the reason of the substitution of the fish for the lamb, which represented the former dispensation.[4]

III

Before entering on the subject of the present letter, I wish to observe concerning it and its predecessor of the last number, that she sole object of the criticisms and interpretations I am now placing before the readers of this Magazine, is to suggest to conscientious Christians a ground of reconciliation between the tenets of their faith and the practice of vegetarianism, so that they may not fancy themselves forced to conclude that religion sanctions and even inculcates that which their own secret sense of morality condemns. It may be that in the course of my exposition I may offend some, who, despite personal conviction and rule of life, yet prefer to abide by the popular exoteric sense attributed to the text of the Old and New Testaments. I beg such to have patience with me for the sake of others, who, like myself, are bent on ***systematising*** their thought, and to whom it is a serious difficulty to be unable to regard the personages whom sacred tradition presents to us as types of perfection, as failing in respect of one of the chief articles in the moral code by which they regulate their own lives.

In my last letter I pointed out some of the many reasons we have for supposing that the fish-eating and marine occupation attributed to Jesus and his Apostles are, as admittedly are many Bible histories, allegorical and mystical in character. And this appears the more probable, when, in support of the facts already adduced, we remember that in Hebrew scripture many passages occur connecting Messiahship and the office of the Prophet of Mercy with the Sea and Fishery; while, on the other hand, the Avenger and the function of the Prophet of Wrath are symbolised under the figures of Hunter and the Arrow. Thus, in ***Jeremiah*** xvi, 16, "Behold, I will send for many fishers, saith the Lord, and they shall fish them; and after I will send for many hunters, and they shall hunt them." And in **_Ezekiel_** xlvii, "There shall be a very great multitude of fish, because the waters shall come thither, for they shall be healed, and everything shall live whither the river cometh. And it shall come to pass that the fishers shall stand over the waters. From Engedi even unto Eneglaim there shall be spreading forth of nets, their fish shall be according to their kinds, as the fish of the great sea, exceeding many." [5] For the net of the Fisher gathers, draws, and encloses, as does the doctrine of the Messiah of Peace, taking men's souls, not by violence, but by the attraction and subtleties of love. But the arrow of the Hunter strikes, wounds, and destroys, as does the vengeance of the Lord by the hand of those whom He appoints to be Ministers of Wrath. The first are the Sons of the Water, or of the Virgin, whose robe in all legendary art is characteristically depicted as blue; the latter are the Sons of the Fire, bearing the flaming sword of justice, and purifying the Earth as fire purifies, not by cleansing but by consuming. The perfect balance and combination of these two colours, blue and red, produces the royal purple, as the perfect harmony of love and justice characterises the Divine King.

The Messiah of the Gospels is thus associated with the sea, and redemption through and by water, as are His prototypes, Noah, Moses, and

Jonah, all of whom were saviours, and messengers of mercy.

It remains to speak of the sense in which, from the vegetarian Christian's point of view, may be understood certain allusions to flesh-eating in the parables recorded by the Evangelists. The most notable of these allusions occurs in the story of the Prodigal Son, on whose return home "the fatted calf" is slain. We may, I think, regard this statement and others of a similar character, – including the account of Peter's vision, [6] – as belonging to a class of illustrations – frequent in both Old and New Testaments – which, though based upon common and popular practices and customs, cannot be taken as intended either to sanction or to perpetuate them. For if such illustrations are to be held commendatory of flesh-eating, we should, on the same ground, be forced to admit that Jesus approved the institution of slavery; since, not only in His own teaching and in that of His apostles, nothing appears against it; but in **Luke** xvii, 9, we find a verse which can hardly be regarded as representing our modern views of what should be the conduct of a Christian master towards his servant. It may be noted also, that the word translated "servant" in this verse, and generally so translated throughout the New Testament, is not μισθωTης – one who serves for hire, – as in the parable of the Prodigal Son, and in **Mark** i, 20; or even οἰκέTης as in

Peter's admonitory address, but **δοῦλος**, – a slave, a bondman. We do not need to be reminded that for many years serious opposition to the Anti-Slavery movement was offered by "religious" persons, on the ground that the inspired writers of both Old and New Testaments not only abstain from condemning the institution of slavery, but even provide codes of laws, penal and otherwise, for regulating the mutual relations of masters and bondmen. Precisely the same observations apply to questions concerning the social position of women, which, in spite of biblical and apostolical restraint, tends every year to grow worthier and nobler. In our times no Christian community exists that would not be ashamed to accept the laws formulated in the Old Testament with regard to marriage, plurality of "wives", the punishment of infidelity in the woman, the relations between parent and child, the conduct of war, the treatment of prisoners, and the like; to none of which, however, do we hear that Jesus took any serious exception. For even in the story of the woman "take in adultery," the law which adjudged her to death by stoning is not condemned, but only its administration by the hands of those present on the occasion. In the same manner modern thought and experience have greatly modified the powers and authority of princes, which at the time of the Apostles were despotic and tyrannous. Yet the principle of this tyranny is nowhere condemned. Instances still more startling may be found in the prophecy of Hosea, who, as a "sign," is twice commanded to commit what Christians would consider a gross offence against morality (**Hosea** i, 2, and iii, 2); in **Kings** xxii, 22, 23, where we find the "Lord" giving a direct sanction to falsehood; in the blessing pronounced on the treacherous and cruel Jael: in the Divine instigation attributed to the act of the murderer Ehud (**Judges** iii, 15), and in analogous cases, too numerous even for mention.

Truth to tell, the "letter" of the scriptures is not that which Christians should regard as itself the veritable "word," for not only is the "letter" in most instances unimportant, but it even "killeth"; that is to say, that, if exclusively venerated, it destroys the reason and the moral conscience. The "spirit" alone it is which "giveth life," and it is precisely this "spirit" of Christ, which is also the spirit of freedom and justice, that has led men step by step to liberate their fellows from hereditary chains and slavery; to curtail the despotism of monarchs; to observe international courtesies in time of war; to spare the families of the vanquished from outrage and murder; to emancipate women from servitude and enforced seclusion, – a work yet far from completion; – and, last and latest, to recognise the rights of dumb beings and the duties their human brethren owe them. The living Christ in man it is who has done and is doing work like this; the Christ-spirit which reforms institutions by first reforming men.

---

1. These *Letters on Pure Diet*, written by Anna Kingsford, first appeared in **The Food Reform Magazine** in the months of July and October 1881, and January 1882, respectively. They were reprinted in **The Ideal in Diet**, which was published in 1898, as vol. ix of the Vegetarian Jubilee Library. The first of these *Letters* was, in part, incorporated by Anna Kingsford in her *Lecture on Food* (p. 77 *post*), and it is reprinted here as revised or added to in such lecture. The second *Letter* was incorporated (almost verbatim) by Anna Kingsford and Edward Maitland in their third article in the controversy, "*The Perfect Way" and its Critics*, in **Light**, in 1882, which followed the publication of their book, **The Perfect Way** (see **Light**, 9th December 1882, p. 551, and *Biographical Preface*, p. 45 *ante*). The second *Letter* is reprinted here as revised or added to in the above-mentioned article in **Light**; and such article has been also reprinted in *Appendix III* of the new (Fourth) Edition of **The Perfect Way**. – S.H.H.
2. The wine used by Jesus at the Last Supper is stated by some authorities to have been **unfermented** grape juice. Those, therefore, who believe that Jesus partook of wine in the **literal** sense, need not assume that Jesus transgressed the rule of his order. Anna Kingsford was of opinion that the connection of Jesus with bread and wine is equally mystic in its character as is that of Jesus with fish and fish-eating, and "needs no explanation for those who are acquainted with the facts and doctrines of ancient mythology and the relation of the latter to the religion of which they are the lineal ancestors" (**Light**, 1882, p. 552).
3. This observation is not less pertinent if we suppose the Fourth Gospel to have been written, not by John, but **according** to John, for in either case it would record his version of the event in question.

4. In a letter dated 11th April 1893, to the Rev. J.G. Ouseley, Edward Maitland, refering to the miracle of the loaves and fishes, says: – "About Jesus eating fish – the Gospels are so mystical that the word 'fish' may well be taken as symbolising the doctrine of Love or mysteries of Aphrodite the Sea-Queen, to whom the fish was sacred; while the loaves would imply the fellow mysteries of Demeter the Earth-Mother. For it was no part of a Christ's mission to provide the materials for a huge physical picnic. The multitude was famished for spiritual sustenance, and the loaves and fishes supplied by him would be of that kind." In other words: as the "loaves" represent "the Lesser Mysteries whose grain is of the Earth"; the "fishes" – which are given after the loaves – imply the Greater Mysteries, the fish being born in the "waters," which are, symbolically, of the Soul and its kingdom. The fish, therefore, represents the interior mysteries of the soul (see **The Perfect Way**, *Lecture VIII*, par. 28; and *Lecture IX*, par. 10).
5. A note on this text in the Douay Version of the **Bible**, says, "These waters are not be understood literally, but mystically, of the baptism of Christ, and of his doctrine and grace; the trees that grow on the banks are Christian virtues; the fishes are Christians, that spiritually live in and by these holy waters; the fishermen are the apostles, and apostolic preachers."
6. The fact that Peter, while he understood the vision as a command to "kill and eat," **refused** to obey the command – a command, be it remembered, thrice uttered, – notwithstanding his hunger and desire to eat, proves, conclusively, that he, like his Master, was, **on principle**, a non-eater of such foods as come within the description of the animals which, in his vision, he saw let down in the sheet, viz.: – "All manner of four-footed beasts, and creeping things of the earth, and fowls of the heaven": a description that embraces and includes the very foods which are abjured by non-flesh eaters. Peter declined to do what he was not in the habit of doing, and what was revolting to his moral nature, and it is not without significance that at the time when he so declined to "kill and

eat" he was "upon the house-top" of his higher consciousness. He was in the place of communion with God. How, in the face of this, Peter's vision can be regarded as an argument in ***favour*** of flesh-eating, I fail to understand. If it should be argued that Peter's vision at least represents God as being in favour of or not against flesh-eating, the answer is: – as Peter's vision, admittedly, was **not** intended as a command to Peter to kill and eat any animal, but to teach him not to call any man common or unclean, it cannot be used to shew that God has ever commanded or that He approves of flesh-eating. – S.H.H.

3. A LECTURE ON FOOD

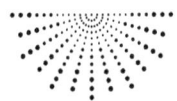

IT[1] requires rather a course of lectures than a lecture to treat adequately, and in all its bearings, the subject upon which you have invited me to address you. For it is one which, being appropriately plant-like in nature, has many root-fibres, which penetrate into various strata of knowledge and experience, and the shadow it casts extends over a vast area of thought, related as well to the future as to the past.

I might, for instance, invite your attention to the consideration of human dietetics in the light of history. I might point to the opening of the Kabbalistic Book of Genesis, the origin of which is undoubtedly Indo-Egyptian, as evidence of the teaching of the sacred mysteries in regard to the nature of the food proper to man in an unfallen state; or I might cite to you the famous passages in which Ovid describes the Golden or Arcadian Age, when, "contented with the food which nature freely gave, men were happy in the fruit of trees, and herbs of earth, nor stained their lips with blood." And I might point out to you further, what also Ovid well shews in the speech he puts into the mouth of the Samian sage; how, with the odious practice of flesh-eating, came likewise that of bloody sacrifice and aggressive war, – a dismal triad, whose mutual relations are nowhere so forcibly and graphically portrayed as in the **Iliad** of Homer. But that I do not desire to weary you with quotations and references, I might remind you of the teachings of that purest and noblest school of Greek philosophy to which Pythagoras gave his name, and which, through the influence of his disciples of a later age, Porphyry and Iamblichus, became the parent of Neo-platonism; I might cite the letters of Seneca to Lucilius; Plutarch's celebrated **Essay on Flesh-Eating**, and certain passages from the **Republic** of Plato, the chief exponent in which dialogue is Socrates; I might speak of Tertullian's treatise on abstinence from animal meats, in which he criticises Paul's observations on the subject; and of works having a similar import from the pens of Clement of Alexandria and Chrysostom the Golden-mouthed. I might recall to your minds the innumerable army of prophets, heroes, saints, hermits, and fathers of both Orient and Occident, whose practice, whether as Magi, Therapeuts, Brahmans, Buddhists, Nazarites, Essenes, Ebionites, or Gnostics, was identical with that of the modern school of Akreophagists. Or, quitting antiquity, I might speak to you of Gassendi, Ray, Cheyne, Antonio Cocchi, Rousseau, Wesley, Nicholson, Lambe, Swedenborg, Gleizes, Graham, Lamartine, Struve, Shelley the king of poets, and many another illustrious or well-remembered name.

But as my time is brief and my theme long, I must content myself with only a scant indication of the witness borne to the doctrines of our School by the great and gifted of bygone and present times, and pass on to touch on a few points of more practical and immediate interest.

I shall say first a few words in relation to the anatomical, physiological, and chemical aspects of human dietetics; next I shall speak of the economical, sanitary, and aesthetic bearings of the question; lastly, I shall give a few suggestions which may help you to formulate a more complete and satisfactory code of social and personal ethics than that commonly enunciated from modern pulpits and platforms.

Whether we adopt the theory of the Evolutionists or that of the Creationists – and I may as well say at the outset that I hold the former, as containing the only intelligible and scientific explanation of natural order and phenomena – we must equally admit the Linnaean classification of animals, by which man is placed in the same series as the Ape family. All the characteristics of the human creature are equally those of the higher Primates, and in particular of the orang-outang, the gorilla, and the chimpanzee. Their cranium, their cerebral convolutions, their teeth and dental morphology, their jaw action and glandular appendages, their stomach, liver, and alimentary canal, their hands adapted for fruit-gathering and tree-climbing – all these, refined and elaborated, are distinctly human in character, and differ in every particular from the carnivorous attributes of predacious beasts on the one hand, and on the other, from those of the ruminant herbivora. Now the Ape family, man included, are all naturally frugivorous. The food of the anthropoids is derived from tree and grain produce, and though some of the tribe are great egg-suckers and insect-hunters, these pursuits are incidental only, and are clearly due, especially as regards the latter, to the curiosity and love of mischief which characterise alike the ape and the savage man. In no zoological collection that I ever yet heard of is the ape or the monkey supplied with any flesh food, or even with animal products. The rations served daily to these creatures in the Jardin des Plantes at Paris, and in the gardens of the Zoological Society of London, consist of rice, potatoes, apples, bread, and salad. Pouchet, Owen, Cuvier, Linné, Lawrence, Bell, Gassendi, and Flourens all agree in attributing a frugivorous nature to man. Flourens says: "Man is neither carnivorous nor herbivorous. He has neither the teeth of the cud-chewers, nor their multiple stomachs, nor their intestines. If we consider these organs in man, we must conclude him to be by nature frugivorous, as is the ape."

Now, the digestive apparatus of the family to which man belongs, may, broadly speaking, be divided into three separate receptacles and laboratories, to each of which a distinct function is appropriated. These three departments are the stomach, the intestines, and the liver, and to each corresponds a special chemical division of alimentary substances, known to modern science respectively as nitrogenous, fatty, and starchy foods. The first-named group, the nitrogenous foods, are fourfold in constitution, containing carbon, hydrogen, oxygen, and nitrogen, with traces of sulphur and phosphorus. Nitrogenised compounds are obtainable from both vegetable and animal sources, and their forms are known as albumen, fibrine, caseine, gelatine, and chondrine. In vegetables they are procurable chiefly from seeds; in animals, from muscular tissue. The first three substances, albumen, fibrine, and caseine, appear primarily in the vegetable kingdom, and are known to chemists as ***proteinaceous*** substances. By this term it is meant that by the action of heat and an alkali these three forms of nitrogenised matter furnish a new substance called proteine, produced in the process by transformation only, and this fact serves to distinguish them from gelatine and chondrine, products of animal origin, which, although nitrogenised, are not capable of yielding proteine. Albumen, fibrine, and caseine, identical in both organic kingdoms as regards nature and properties, differ slightly from one another. **Albumen** contains a considerable proportion of sulphur and phosphorus, and exists in both the soluble and the coagulated state, the latter condition being due to the application of heat above the ordinary temperature. It forms the substance known as "white of egg," which when raw is fluid, and becomes solid by being subjected to a process of cooking. It is contained in all the cereals, in all seeds, and in the juices of most herbaceous vegetables. **Fibrine** differs from albumen by its characteristic tenaciousness, and by the fact that it coagulates without heat. More sulphur is present in fibrine than in albumen. In the animal system fibrine is the material which forms the basis of muscular tissue and the thickening substance of the blood. In vegetables it constitutes the basis of gluten – the firm portion of seeds and grains. **Caseine** neither coagulates spontaneously, as does fibrine, nor by heat, as does albumen. It contains sulphur, but no phosphorus. It is obtainable from milk, and therefore from all milky compounds, and from all peas, beans, and other leguminous seeds.

Not long ago the view taken by scientific men

of the uses of proteinaceous food was a very different one from that which recent observation and inquiry seem to have satisfactorily established as correct. In accordance with Liebig's hypothesis, nitrogenous (or proteine-giving) material used to be regarded as the only and exclusive source of muscular and nervous ***power***. It was held that nitrogenous matter, after becoming incorporated with muscular tissue and passing through that condition, disintegrated in the system into two constituent parts, one of which was eliminated from the body as waste material, and the other retained for the production of heat and energy. Thus, it was thought, all food must become ***organised tissue*** before it can contribute to force production; and the tissues of the body being consumed in the manifestation of functional activity, and exhausted by metamorphosis into force, nitrogenous matter must be constantly ingested to replace the double loss and expenditure involved. Although ***partially*** true, this hypothesis erred in attributing to nitrogenised food the work of supply of power as well as of repair of tissue. In fact, the force evolved by muscular action does not, as Liebig supposed, proceed from destruction of muscular tissue; his assumption to this effect having been abundantly disproved by the analysis of the effete matters thrown off from the system during muscular exertion, and by careful research undertaken by numerous investigators, and based both on experiment and on arithmetical calculation. The truth appears to be that the property of proteinaceous foods is pre-eminently to serve as material for the development and for the renovation of the various tissues and secretions of the economy. As waste is perpetually occurring alike in muscular, nervous, and glandular tissue, and as a vast quantity of secreted juices is constantly expended in the work of the vital processes, it is of great importance that nitrogenous aliment sufficient to compensate these losses, and to repair the substantial elements of the economy, should be ingested daily.

All the various groups of nitrogenous food are digested in the stomach by means of the gastric juice, a secretion having an acid reaction, and of which the active elements are a soluble ferment called pepsine – whereby albuminous foods are converted into peptones – and an acid, closely resembling in nature and characteristics the mineral product known as hydrochloric or muriatic acid. The effects of the gastric juice on the three chief groups of nitrogenous food, viz., albumen, fibrine, and caseine, differ slightly in detail, but under its influence **all** are liquefied, dissolved, transformed, and rendered fit for assimilation. This digestive process is greatly aided by animal heat, and by the mechanical action set up during the operation in the muscular walls of the organ itself, which, like every other organ of the living body, is intelligent in its functions and takes an active part in the offices of life. From the stomach, the liquefied food, or chyme, is passed on into the next digestive department, where, if necessary, it is further elaborated, and in which the process of absorption commences.

The nitrogenised foods in ordinary use in this country are more commonly derived from the animal than from the vegetable kingdom. They comprise milk and cheese, eggs, lean flesh-meats, poultry, game, and fish; beans, haricots, peas, lentils, all the cereals, nuts, and some herbs. Of these various materials, the proportion of nitrogen yielded by flesh, poultry, game, and fish is much less than that yielded by an equal percentage of cheese and vegetable matter. Beef and mutton, for instance, give an average of 18 %, of nitrogen; pork and ham, 8 %; white fish, 17 %; while cheeses range in nitrogenous value from 25 to 44 %, and the bean tribe from 25 to 30 %. There is thus, ***a priori***, a greater advantage in nitrogenous value to be derived from a given amount of vegetable and milk food than from the same amount of flesh meat. But there is another consideration, important to the ***human*** being who desires not only that his food should be nutritious but that it should be ***pure***. Comestibles of every kind, and nitrogenised foods in particular, contain, besides nutritive matter, elements improper to assimilation, and destined to be rejected by the economy as waste or "ash." These elements are divisible into two categories: substances innutritious by their nature but not impure or vitiated in constitution, such as cellulose, and the woody fibre of plants and all ***vegetable*** products; and substances both innutritious and vitiated, such as are contained in the juices of flesh meats.

The finest and healthiest animal tissue is always permeated by blood, for it is impossible, unless by processes which would utterly ruin it as food, to separate blood from the solid material everywhere pervaded by the circulating vessels. Flesh and blood are therefore virtually inseparable, and their component elements are continually interchanging. Now, as the blood is the vehicle of the sewage of the body, as well as the medium of reconstitution, it contains always two kinds of materials, of which part represents nutrition and part impurity and decomposition. In eating animal flesh, we consume, therefore, as well as the healthy and nutritive matter momentarily fixed in the tissue, certain substances in course of expulsion, decaying products returning into the blood, and destined for elimination from the body of the animal by the various channels appropriated to waste residue. These matters, in process of "retrograde metamorphosis," are known to chemists by such names as creatine, creatinine, xanthine, protagon, tyrosine, sarcosine, inosic, formic, and butyric acids, and so forth.

I do not now speak of the innumerable perils and disgusting associations connected with the eating of **diseased** flesh. These will be touched on when we come to the sanitary considerations of our subject. I desire in this place to point out what impurities and degenerate products are ***inevitably*** consumed by every kreophagist, be he never so fastidious, careful, or delicately served.

As the stomach is physiologically related to the digestion of nitrogenous compounds, so are the intestine and the liver to that of fatty and starchy foods. These foods differ from nitrogenous aliments in their constitution, which, instead of being fourfold, comprise three elements only – carbon, hydrogen, and oxygen. The fatty substances are called by chemists, hydro-carbons; and the starches and sugars, carbo-hydrates. The first group contains carbon, hydrogen, and a ***small*** amount of oxygen; the second comprises carbon, with hydrogen and oxygen in the exact proportion of two volumes of hydrogen to one of oxygen, H_2O – the formula of water. To the hydro-carbons belong all the vegetable oils, yielded by seeds, nuts, stems, etc., and all the animal fats – butter, lard, suet, and dripping. To the carbo-hydrates belong substances obtainable – with one single exception – only from the vegetable kingdom – starch, sugar, gum, fruit-jelly, and cellulose.

Modern experimentation in physics, aided by the application of chemical analysis, has demonstrated that as nitrogenous food corresponds to the development and renovation of living material, so carbonaceous food, of both groups above named, corresponds to the production in the living organism of heat, and consequently of force, – heat and force being mutually convertible. And although, from a chemical point of view, it is necessary to distinguish between the hydro-carbons and the carbo-hydrates – the proportion of oxygen being uniformly larger in the latter than in the former – the physiological uses and character of the two groups may be said to be identical. Both pass through the stomach without change, both are digested in the small intestine, both appear to be finally assimilated under the same form, and both are charged with the function of heat and force production.

Fatty substances – hydro-carbons – consist chemically of a principle possessing acid properties, called fatty acid, in combination with a **radical**. A "radical" in chemical language is a composite body forming a molecular group capable of acting as a simple body in combination, and transferable from one combination to another in exchange for one or more atoms of hydrogen or its representatives. Fats, under which head, of course, oils are included, are decomposed by alkalies, and by certain ferments contained in the juices of the small intestine. These juices are three in number, – the intestinal, secreted by the small glands of the intestine itself; the pancreatic, secreted by the pancreas; and the bile, secreted by the liver. The last-named secretion, however, appears to take no active part in digestion; and although physiologists have long disputed its function, the general tendency now is to regard it as destined to play the part rather of scullion than of cook in the culinary department in which it officiates. That is to say, that while the process of digestion is going on in the intestine, the bile does not arrive on the scene at all; but when the work of the other juices is pretty nearly finished – when the endothelium or superficial cells which line the intestine and take part in the act of absorption, have begun to peel off and decorticate – then the bile flows in, sweeps away these deteriorated cells, cleans down the whole laboratory, renews its surface, and puts everything in order for new work. Thus it prevents putrid fermentation of the intestinal contents, and repairs the mucous lining of the alimentary canal. But to the intestinal glandular secretion, and especially to the pancreatic juice, is committed the operation of the digestive process. The main part of this process, the emulsification of all the fats and oils, is performed almost exclusively by the pancreatic juice, an alkaline secretion which flows into the intestine immediately on the arrival of the food, and of which the active principle is a mixture of three particular ferments. The fat is thus broken up, and parted into very minute globules, such as are contained in milk, and in this condition it is sucked up and absorbed by the little cellular projecting tubes which line the intestine. Upon starch and other amyloid matters, comprised under the term carbo-hydrates, and belonging therefore to the second group of non-nitrogenised solid foods, the action of the intestinal juices is equally strong. Although these are destined to undergo their final transformation elsewhere, it is in the intestine that they become converted into sugar, which, passing by virtue of its diffusibility into the circulating current of the blood-vessels, is thus conveyed by the portal system into the liver. It is not precisely determined by what physiological process this saccharine matter eventually becomes absorbable by the organism, but that the process, whatever its details, takes place in the liver, and that it is ultimately in the form of fatty matter that all sugary material is utilised in the human body, appear, according to modern writers, to be indubitable facts.

Of hydro-carbons or fats, the most valuable, but unfortunately the least known and used in this country, are derived from vegetable sources. These are much more digestible and suitable food than the animal fats, partly on account of the assured purity and freedom from disease of their origin, and partly on account of their more sound and wholesome nature, less liable to decomposition and alteration than fats obtained from beasts. The best-known vegetable oil is that of the olive, procured from the fruit by pressure. In France this oil is largely replaced by **huile d'oliette**, expressed from poppy seeds, and which, being tasteless, is most valuable for cooking purposes. The seeds of the sunflower yield 40 % of oil, and oils of very fine quality are also procurable in large quantities from linseed, cotton-seed, mustard-seed, rape-seed, sesamum, the seeds of the common cucumber, and other grains. Seed-oils are largely used in the East, where the national religious customs preclude the use of animal fats. Palm oil is, like olive oil, a fruit product, and is obtained from the pericarp of a palm-tree growing in tropical Africa. All nuts, of whatever kind, contain oil in large quantities, and some, as the almond and cocoa nut, are extensively used in commerce for the sake of their richness in this respect. **Solid** vegetable oils, or butter, are procurable from several species of Indian and African plants. The seeds of the Indian "butter-tree" contain a substance which in the fresh state resembles animal butter, but which hardens gradually, and becomes suet-like in consistence. "This butter," says Mungo Park, in his ***Travels in Africa***, "besides the advantage of keeping sweet the whole year round without salt, is whiter, firmer, and to my taste, of a richer flavour than the best butter made from cow's milk." Dr. Pavy tells us that the growth and preparation of this commodity seem to be among the first objects of African industry, and to constitute a main article of the national commerce.

The carbo-hydrates, with one single exception only, come to us from the vegetable kingdom. The exception is lactine, or sugar of milk. True, a substance analogous to starch is found in the liver, and under certain diseased conditions in flesh tissue, but for alimentary purposes these sources are not available. Sugar is of three kinds: milk-sugar (just named), cane-sugar – the crystallised variety in common use, extracted from stems and roots – and grape-sugar, procurable from every kind of fruit. Honey is also a vegetable product, being collected from flowers by the insects whose food it is. It appears that in the living human organism sugar is more readily assimilable than most substances; and if the deductions of physiologists are trustworthy, it plays so necessary a part in vital processes, that, as Dr. Edward Smith observes, "it may be doubted whether the loss of any one element of food would be so keenly felt as that of sugar. It enters universally into the dietaries of every class of mankind in every place." In fact, physiology has demonstrated that **grape** sugar, under which form **cane** sugar and all saccharine compounds are assimilated, performs in the living body certain indispensable functions beyond that of heat and force production. It excites and assists the digestive processes, furnishes abundant chyle, and probably stimulates the secretion of the salivary glands, always more copious and necessary in fruit and grain-eating animals than in predaceous mammals. Dr. Playfair, in his dietaries, while allotting to nitrogenous matter a proportion of four ounces only, and to fatty substances two ounces, considers carbo-hydrates – starch and sugar – necessary to the extent of seventeen or eighteen ounces daily.

Starchy substances are usually described as farinaceous foods. The articles of this nature chiefly in use among us are sago, tapioca, cassava, arrowroot, potato, semolina, rice, vermicelli, maccaroni, and all the meals and beans generally. It must be borne in mind that these foods, especially the corn and bean-meals, represent also the prime sources of nitrogenous food. Dry common wheat contains on an average 77 % of hydrates of carbon, and from 15 to 20 % of nitrogenous material. Barley-meal, rye-meal, quinoa-meal, buckwheat, maize, and oatmeal give an average of about 70 % of carbo-hydrates and 12 of nitrogen, the rest being made up of oily matter and salts.

The type of all human foods – bread – comes to us from the vegetable world, and the fact that this aliment is popularly regarded as the "staff of life," and the poetical equivalent of all possible forms of nutritive matter, is in perfect accord with the estimate of science; for as fruit, or grain – which botanically are identical – is the most highly vitalised, solarised, pure, and essential product of organic life, so the food which is composed of grain is the most precious to the human economy. In the wheat-grain are contained all the elements necessary for the fulfilment of the twofold function of alimentation of which I have already spoken. The cells of the central part of the grain contain starch, whereby are produced force and heat; the cells underlying the husk contain nitrogenous substance, whereby tissues are built up; and in the outer sheathings are found the phosphates and other mineral materials which enter into the constitution of the animal economy. The wheat-grain is thus a microcosmic epitome of the various classes of food with which physiological chemistry has made us acquainted.

Thus it is obvious that from the vegetable kingdom are derived the best and purest forms of human alimentation. This kingdom not only supplies us abundantly with the agents of heat and labour, the animal sources of which are totally inadequate to meet our needs, but it yields us also food of a nitrogenous character, infinitely healthier, more cleanly, and richer in value than the flesh of any beast or fowl. For these reasons among many others, it seems evident that in the operations of normal evolution, plant-life must everywhere precede animal-life; and that the carnivorous groups of the latter are to be regarded rather as the result of a degradation from, or retrogression in, the process of natural development – due to incidental disasters – than as the outcome of its orderly march.

I have not time, in view of the many important subjects which press for consideration, to enter upon the question of the relation of food to national resources. It is a question of profound interest and import to the political economist, the farmer, the landlord, the peasant-tenant, and the philanthropic reformer, and needs a treatise to expound its manifold bearings. But, leaving this momentous subject untouched, the question of food economy is interesting from a social and domestic, as well as from a national point of view. A great part of the burden of poverty, which in most of our large centres presses so severely on the labouring classes, would be removed were a cheaper system of diet introduced into their homes. It has just been shewn that many inexpensive kinds of vegetable food contain a percentage of nutritive material, both nitrogenous and carbonaceous, greatly exceeding that which can be obtained from costly joints of flesh-meat, the waste of which in cooking averages from a third to half the original weight. An outlay of a shilling in oatmeal, peas, lentils, or beans will purchase as much nutriment as five shillings expended on butcher's meat. An idea of the immense economy which might be effected by a more judicious use and distribution of food-stuffs than that at present in vogue, may be gathered from Mr. Hoyle's computation, that if the six million families of the United Kingdom were to reduce their consumption of butcher's meat by a pound's weight only a week, it would give a saving of ten or more million pounds sterling per annum.

If there be a moral lesson to be got out of statistics relating to domestic expenditure, it is one which pre-eminently concerns our national school boards. Let the authorities who hold in their hands the guidance of the rising generation, and therefore the immediate future of the country, take up the question of food-supply and domestic economy in a practical form, and teach the boys and girls committed to their care how to make the most out of the wages they will earn when they grow to be men and women. Let the children of the people be taught the values of food-stuffs, and the elements of organic chemistry – a kind of learning which would be of far more practical service to them than much of that which the "standards" now require, and the results of which would, in the best sense, be productive of civilisation and prosperity. And let attention, moreover, be given to the instruction of the girls in the science and resources of housekeeping, with special reference to the neglected art of vegetable cookery, and of making savoury and appetising dishes out of inexpensive materials. As a rule, the poor, and even the middle classes, in England have no idea of cookery as applied to any other material than animal meats. Boiled potatoes and cabbage, or potatoes "baked under the joint," express the limit of the popular notions with regard to vegetable comestibles. And in proportion to the restriction of their resources in this respect the people's health and purses suffer.

There is far greater perspicacity and economy shewn with regard to the choice of foods among the peasant classes on the Continent. In Switzerland, Germany, Norway, Italy, Spain, Holland, Belgium, and France, flesh-meat is rarely seen on the tables of agricultural labourers, and the omelette, the homemade cheese, the maccaroni stew, the **olla podrida**, the **pot-au-feu** take the place of the indigestible joint of pork, the steak pie, or the uncleanly tripe, which in this country consume the family earnings and preclude expenditure upon real necessities. For need of the proper instruction, which might be given in the national schools, but of which, alas! the instructors themselves stand in need, the poor are universally impressed with the belief that the prime source of all nourishment worth the name is to be found in butcher's meat, and to obtain this desideratum they will sacrifice in one day a sum which, spent with knowledge, would suffice for a week's comfort.

It is not by taking yearly more of our home lands from tillage and labour and laying them waste for rearing cattle that we shall increase either national prosperity or the material welfare of families. Such means as these carry with them three inevitable and direct evil tendencies, of which the first is to increase the chances of cattle epidemics by overstocking, and by the artificial feeding and rearing of farm-beasts for the market, – both fruitful sources of peril, especially as regards the production of entozoa, or worm affections, the varieties of which among stall-fed animals are very great. The second evil tendency is to throw out of work a large number of agricultural labourers, and to depopulate the country by diminution of the quantity of available food produced, thus fostering distress and bringing about enforced emigration. And the third evil consists in the multiplication of slaughter-houses, meat-markets, depots for offal and hides, tanneries, and many offensive and unhealthy trades connected with the butcher's avocation in and near large cities, thereby detracting enormously from the beauties and pleasures of civilised life, and increasing proportionately its discomforts, and the risks of infectious fevers, zymotic contagion, and diseases arising from the decomposition of animal matter.

We thus come to the consideration of a few facts related to the sanitary aspect of kreophagy.

Dr. Creighton, addressing the Medical Congress of 1881 on the subject of "*Diseases communicated to Man by the Meat and Milk Supply*," said: –

"One ground of our alarm on this subject is that tubercle – or, as it is called, pearl disease – is quite common in the species of animals to which we trust so implicitly – one might almost say, so blindly – for a large part of our food. (...) The disease is inherited and chronic, and may be present for years in the body of an animal and give rise to no symptoms. The distinctive formations of the disease are sometimes found in animals that have been slaughtered in (apparently) perfect condition. But the disease in its worst form (...) is mostly met with in milch cows. (...) The cow-houses in or near large towns are said to contain the largest proportion of diseased animals; the close confinement throughout the whole year, the artificial food, the want of fresh air and of sunlight, all tending to bring out the disease. The cows are milked as long as it is profitable to milk them, and they are then sold out of the herd, probably to the butcher. (...) Without adopting alarmist estimates (...) there need be no hesitation in concluding that the milk of cows in a more or less advanced state of tubercular disease is constantly being consumed both by infants and by adults. (...) As for the flesh, there are the lymphatic glands and viscera, and inferior parts of the carcase, such as the diaphragm, or 'skirt,' which are especially liable to have the actual tubercular nodules adhering to them, or more or less intimately blended with them. These inferior parts of the animal are sold at a cheap rate to the poor, and there is neither popular prejudice nor legislative enactment to hinder the tubercular meat from being sold. (...) Two days ago I sent a trustworthy person to certain slaughter-houses in London, with instructions to bring me specimens of pearl nodules from as many animals as he could find. He brought specimens from four old cows which were slaughtered in his presence. The lungs were riddled with purulent cavities; the meat would be sold at about fourpence a pound to be made into sausages and saveloys. There is, then, no doubt at all that the species of domestic animals which is so much in our confidence that we drink of one of its secretions, and eat of its flesh, and even of its viscera, is a species that is widely tainted with tubercular disease. That alone is fact enough to cause uneasiness. (...) On the 22nd of July 1881, I took the opportunity of attending a meeting of the National Veterinary Congress, and heard from a veterinary surgeon of Peterborough a narrative which brought out the value of our present evidence. A cow, which he knew professionally to be in an advanced state of tuberculosis, was sold out of a large farm for £5; the purchaser kept the cow for the exclusive supply of his family with milk and butter. Since then, the man's wife and one of his children had died of rapid consumption, and the man himself was now also dying of the same disease."

In the course of the discussion which followed

Dr. Creighton's paper, Dr. A. Carpenter observed that it had been shown by "evidence given in a court of law that ninety % of the animals which were slaughtered for the Metropolitan Meat Market were more or less infected with tubercle. It was shown too that this was almost universally the case in cows which had become barren. (...) Meat and milk from diseased beasts could not be healthy; and so long as animals were kept in close, ill-ventilated sheds, disease would abound among them. The time must come," he thought, "when they would be kept in the manner which nature designed them to be, viz. in the open fields of the country only."

This last remark of Dr. A. Carpenter is certainly sagacious, but it necessarily assumes a vast reduction in the quantity of flesh-meat and milk consumed. For the "open" pastures of this country would not support enough cattle in the "natural" condition of which he speaks to meet a fifth part of the present demand for animal food.

In the same section of the Congress, Mr. F. Vacher presented an address on "*The Influence of Various Articles of Food in spreading Parasitic, Zymotic, Tubercular, and other Diseases.*" Corroborating Dr. Creighton, he said: —

"The foods which alone can spread their own diseases to the subjects by whom they are ingested are necessarily meat and milk, or their derivatives. There is abundant evidence in support of the view that foot-and-mouth disease may be spread to the human subject by means of milk, also tubercle: and as regards meat, there is evidence that a specific disease may be communicated to man by the ingestion of meat tainted with splenic fever or anthracoid disease, and erysipelas (a common symptom in many animal diseases) may spread to man by means of flesh. (...) Other diseases can be spread by means of meat infected by entozoa." [2]

Mr. Ernest Hart, in a long and careful paper, fortified by copious statistics, proved that typhoid fever, scarlatina, and diphteria had been all largely propagated by the use of milk.

"There is nothing," he said, "in the analogy of epidemics to limit the list to these three maladies, and already we are seeing indications of other cognate diseases being spread by the same agency. The number of epidemics of typhoid fever recorded in the abstract as due to milk is fifty; of scarlatina, fifteen; and of diphtheria, seven. The total number of cases during the epidemics traced to the use of infected milk may be reckoned in round numbers as 3500 of typhoid fever, 800 of scarlet fever, and 500 of diphtheria. When it is remembered that barely ten years ago we were utterly ignorant that milk was a carrier of infection, and that all these observations have been taken within one short decade, it will be seen how vitally important is the safe-guarding of our milk supplies from contamination. That so common an article of food as milk should be so readily capable of absorbing infection is a question of greatest moment. The houses invaded during these epidemics were found to be commonly of the better class, and in healthy situations. The poor, who take very little milk, and that only in tea or coffee, generally escaped."

Entozoic diseases, due to the presence in various parts of the body of small parasites – some varieties of which are microscopic – are largely communicable to man, and the consequence of eating the flesh of animals so affected is often fatal, especially in the case of the common pork malady known as **trichinosis**. The large tapeworm, or **taenia**, which in the intestinal cavity of man often acquires a length of many feet, is derived from the bullock, the calf, and the pig; fluke, or liver-worm, is common in the sheep. Usually, in thickly populated districts, the livers of all sheep supplying the markets are riddled with these small worms.

In connection with this part of my subject, I should like to offer a few remarks in regard to the new method of "inoculation" as a preservative against certain forms of cattle and sheep disease. As you are aware, this method, to which Pasteur has attached his name, consists of the introduction into the blood of healthy animals of the attenuated or "cultivated" virus of anthrax, a malignant disease which for some time past has occasionally attacked districts devoted to the rearing of herds and flocks. Now, Pasteurism is the means by which modern science seeks to combat Nature's determination to put down redundant numbers, and to maintain a just equilibrium. Man, for purposes at once unnatural and immoral, has artificially multiplied to an enormous extent certain species of animals, and has given up to their support vast areas of otherwise serviceable land. Whenever any particular kind of animal, not excepting man himself, increases beyond a certain ratio over a limited area, Nature provides means to check the increase, and to restore the balance of species. The flesh-eating propensities of all classes of mankind have, during the last few decades, been steadily growing, and to minister to these propensities domesticated eatable animals have been bred all over the western half of the world in incredible numbers. Cause has brought about effect; overcrowding, artificial living, the impossibility of maintaining invariable sanitary conditions, and other inconveniences connected with breeding, have produced their inevitable nemesis. Pasteur proposes to get the better of Nature by anticipating her hand, and by infecting the yet unsmitten cattle and sheep with a mild form of disease, which shall prevent them from succumbing to its deadlier type. This means simply that so long as the animals are under the influence of the disease, whether mild or malignant, they will not be liable to contract a fresh bout of it. If a person has small-pox in his economy, he will not be liable to any fresh contagion from extraneous sources. But there comes a time, perhaps in seven years or less, perhaps in ten or more – in some persons much sooner – when the influence of the disease will have wholly passed out of the economy, and then the body again becomes liable to contagion. So it is with anthrax in cattle. Pasteur and his followers know this, and they recommend therefore re-inoculations at certain intervals. All of which means that in order to keep our flocks and herds from diminishing, and to be able to meet the unnatural demand for abundance of flesh, and to eat oxen and sheep without stint, we must keep them in a constant state of splenic infection. For be sure that so long as they are "protected," as it is called, so long the deadly **bacillus anthracis** is somewhere about in the tissues and humours of the inoculated animal. Were it not, the "protection" would cease. The system is based on the principle of setting a thief in the house to keep other thieves out. But when once the house-keeping thief departs and leaves the house clean of his presence, the gang outside are liable to break in. Nor is the **bacillus anthracis**, even when fully in possession of the economy, able to keep out other diseases. On the contrary, an official report recently made to the Hungarian Department of Public Health on Pasteur's inoculation declares that "deaths from other complaints, such as catarrh, pneumonia, pericarditis, etc., occurred **exclusively** amongst the inoculated. It follows from this that a fatal issue from other severe diseases is accelerated by protective inoculation." Of this fact also Pasteur and his school are aware, for they now recommend, as Mr. Fleming informs us in the **Nineteenth Century**, the application of the "protective" method to **all** infectious forms of disease! All the zymotic diseases are believed to be inoculable by means of their special bacilli, and it is gravely argued, nay, even urged with all the pompous air of scientific authority, that henceforth the blood of both man and beast should be infected by every one of these germs, and thus be maintained in a continual state of ferment and impurity. "Disease is king," cry the scientists; "long live Disease!" Truly, we may despair of successfully eradicating by means of hygiene and sanitation the myriad forms of living dirt, while "prophylactic medicine," as it is sarcastically termed, industriously multiplies, preserves, circulates, transmits, and sows the fatal germs broadcast over all the earth.

There is, besides, another grave consideration connected with Pasteurism, and one which is specially related to our subject. We have seen how transmissible from cattle to man by means of milk and meat are tubercular disease, foot-and-mouth disease, and other complaints. Why not then splenic disease in similar fashion? Anthrax is communicable to wool-sorters and tanners by mere contact with infected hides; what warrant have we that the secretion and flesh of creatures suffering under the influence of attenuated virus will prove harmless eating and drinking? Such ingesta may not perhaps set up true anthrax, but might develop unpleasant blood-symptoms, and predispose to such diseases as erysipelas, septicaemia, cutaneous eruptions, inflammatory tendencies, or general ill-defined morbid conditions. On this subject the Hungarian Report says: —

"When we consider that the inoculative material contains anthrax microzymes in colossal quantities, although of diminished virulence, and that the microzymes multiply to a gigantic extent in the organism of the inoculated animals, we see that the general employment of protective inoculations would spread these germs in inconceivable quantities through the whole country. Deaths will occur at all times, even among the inoculated animals, and the possibility is not excluded that the microzymes which would be liberated from the dead bodies when they became scattered, might regain their original virulence, and thus, despite all trouble and cost, attack both men and animals. This is all the more to be feared, as the carelessness with which people even now treat the bodies of animals which have died from anthrax would then be increased by belief in the omnipotence of protective inoculation."

So far, I have briefly placed before you a few arguments drawn from comparative anatomy, chemistry, physiology, domestic economy, and hygiene. All these considerations belong to the utilitarian aspects of the subject, and affect us rather as physical than as spiritual beings. But the cause of akreophagy may be pleaded yet more strongly from a higher and distinctly **human** point of view, intimately related to the arts which beautify life and civilise our race, and, better and worthier still than these, to those just, compassionate, and gentle instincts of man, in virtue of which alone he *is* man, differing from and surpassing all other creatures. [3] (...)

Ouida, the novelist, who has contributed to the **Gentleman's Magazine** a very good article against vivisection, writes thus in regard to the practice of flesh-eating.

[Here the lecturer read the passage quoted by her in the first of her *Letters on Pure Diet* in **The Food Reform Magazine**.]

To those of us who have lifted the veil which polite society in general finds it convenient to draw between the fashionable dining-room and the slaughter-house, it is no longer possible to sit down with placid mind and complacent face to a table loaded with carcases, and to bend piously forward while the stereotyped "grace" is mur-

mured, and the Lord is thanked for the mercies graciously bestowed on the carnivorous company! "The ***mercies***!" Heaven save the mark! But the Vegetarian host and his guests have no cause for shame. Their lentils, their rice, their fruits, their savoury dishes have been bought at no cost of suffering, terror, despair, or degradation to man or beast. The gardener, the agriculturist, the reaper, the fruit-gatherer are all of them in the enjoyment of healthy, invigorating, and ennobling pursuits. No odours of blood or death pollute the air they daily breathe, nor do hideous spectacles of pain and carnage occupy their sight from morn to night, and quench for them all the manifold loveliness and sweetness of life. The aroma of fields, of vineyards, of orchards, accompanies the beautiful repast of the man whose meal is such as Nature prompts; but over the banquet of the eater of dead flesh hangs the filthy smell of the shambles.

We are told that great things in the interests of progress, enlightenment, and other sacred names, are being done for the present generation by means of compulsory education and the facilities everywhere provided for instruction in science and literature. We are told that among all classes of the people knowledge is to be increased, intellect cultivated, and civilisation spread. But if, as seems too probable, the chariot of popular education is to be made a vehicle for the propaganda of flesh-eating and vivisection, it will prove but a car of

Juggernaut, whose wheels will assuredly crush the heart out of the people. A system of education merely intellectual tends not to civilise, but to bewilder and to harden. It is idle to speak of "civilising" the children of the new generation by such means as those provided by the Paul Berts of the day, and by others of the modern school of materialistic biology. Education, if it is to be really humanising, refining, and elevating in its results, must be moral and spiritual as well as intellectual. And such an education as this will never be given by men who inculcate on human beings the diet of the tiger, and who teach science by the method of the Spanish Inquisition. Flesh-eating and vivisection are in principle closely related, and both are defended by their advocates on common premises, of which the catch-cries are Utility and the Law of Nature.

As regards the consumption of flesh, it has been shown that being unsuited to the structure and organs of man, comparatively innutritious, largely impure and unsafe, and extremely costly, it certainly cannot be recommended on utilitarian grounds. And in respect to vivisection, though it would be passing strange if a practice carried on throughout Europe for the past two thousand years had effected nothing, its scanty uses have been dearly bought indeed at the cost of the agony involved, and of the rare waste of time, of talent, industry, and intellect over a method mostly vague and futile in its results, other infinitely more exact and valuable means of research being meanwhile neglected. And if such low utilities be veritably of paramount import in the evolution of the race, why have not the vivisectors the courage of their opinions, and why should they not claim – what their arguments legitimately cover – the right to vivisect human creatures? Why, while admitting the principle of vicarious sacrifice, should they shrink from its logical outcome? Is it because of the foolish popular notion that man only has a "soul," while other animals have not? All the more reason then, surely, for sparing these in their one brief life the infliction of suffering which Nature does not impose. Man, with eternity before him, may well afford, for the good of his kind, a few hours or even days of suffering. It is, however, the strange fact that the most atrocious of laboratory tortures are inflicted by men who profess to believe the nature and destiny of the brute and of man identical, and who hold that for both, death is the irrevocable finale of being. From the point of view of this doctrine – a doctrine rapidly gaining power, numbers, and importance in Europe – it is not less difficult to conceive why the brain of the ape should be deemed a fitting object for experiment, and that of the human infant or savage should be spared; why the innocent and serviceable horse or dog should be given over to the tormentors, and the criminal, lunatic, idiot, or pauper should be respected.

As to the second contention, that Nature's law is the law of prey, and that therefore man has ***a priori*** a natural right to rend and torment, it should be answered that the term "Nature" implies neither individuality nor responsibility, but simply **condition**. All that Nature does is to permit the manifestation of acquired qualities ***in individuals***. In such sense we must understand the phrase "habit is Nature." This fact does not justify responsible humanity in the manifestation of cruelties which put to shame the worst of the carnivora. It is by dint of following what Mr. Matthew Arnold calls "the stream of tendency which makes for righteousness" that man has risen out of the baser elements of his nature to the recognition of the standard known as the "golden rule." And it is precisely in proportion as he has set himself, on every plane of his activity, to

*"Move upward, working out
    the beast,
And let the wolf and tiger die"*

within him, that he has become higher, nobler, – in a word, more manly. The modern advocates of flesh-eating and vivisection, on the contrary, would reverse the sentiment of the lines just quoted, and would have us

> *"Move down, returning to the beast,*
> *And letting heart and conscience die,"*

making thereby the practice of the lowest in the scale of Nature the rule of the highest, and abasing the moral standard of mankind to the level of the habits of the most dangerous or noxious orders of brutes.

Our opponents are fond of calling arguments such as these "sentimental," and seem to imagine that the word completely disposes of their value. But that this should be the case serves but to reveal more clearly their own position. For it shows either that they are ignorant of what the word "sentiment" means – ignorant that honour is a sentiment, that courage, truthfulness, love, sympathy, friendship, and every moral quality, the possession of which constitutes the superiority of civilised man over the savage and the brute, are sentiments; or else that they deliberately intend to obliterate these qualities from the curriculum of future generations of mankind, and to exclude them from their definition of humanity. The pretence of modern civilisation is to aim only at the acquirement of intellectual knowledge and physical gratification, with but scant, if any, regard to moral limits. In the creed of the nineteenth century man is man, not because he has it in him to love justice and to refrain from doing wrong, but because, being a pre-eminently clever beast, he is the strongest and most successful of all beasts.

But the disciple of Buddha and of Pythagoras, the preacher of the Pure Life and of the Perfect Way, cries to humanity, "Be men, not in mere physical form only – for form is worth nothing – but in spirit, by virtue of those qualities which exalt you above tigers, swine, or jackals! Under all your pseudo-civilisation lies a foul and festering sore, a moral blemish, staining your lives, and making social amenities unlovely. For the sake of ministering to your depraved and unnatural appetites, there exists a whole class of men, deprived of human rights, whose daily work is to kill, and who pass all their years in shedding blood and in superintending violent death. Away, then, with the slaughter-houses! Make to yourselves a nobler ideal of life and of human destiny!"

To appreciate and comprehend fully the spirit of Vegetarianism, to explain the enthusiasm with which it inspires its professors, a man must be at heart a poet. By this word "poet" I indicate that order of mind which sees intuitively; which seeks Beauty and Perfection as the end of all study and organisation; which formulates a clear Ideal, and makes it everywhere the criterion and guide, as did the Hebrews the Pillar of Flame in the wilderness. Only one of such mind, capable of knowing the Ideal, and of sacrificing all lower attractions to the love of the highest, is able fully to understand the enthusiasm of the Pythagorean, the Buddhist, the abstainer from flesh; the gratification of being innocent of blood-guiltiness, – of knowing that no corpses strew the way to Paradise; and that when voice or pen is employed against cruelty, against oppression, against any one of the many forms of injustice rife among men under the reign of Physical Force, no mortal adversary, no inward conscience can reproach the reformer himself with the daily sacrifice of innocent victims to the false gods of bodily appetite.

Long since, one who has been called the king of poets, Shelley – the sweetest, because the tenderest of singers – in a poem [4] which most of us know as the sustained and earnest protest of a just soul against all modes of tyranny, wrote these words, so pregnant with power and wise love that they seem almost the utterance of a prophetic spirit, foreseeing in a vision the far-off light of the Perfect Day that shall be when the Kingdom of God shall come:

> *"My brethren, we are free!*
> *The fruits are glowing*
> *Beneath the stars, and the*
> *   night winds are flowing*
> *O'er the ripe corn, the birds*
> *   and beasts are dreaming –*

*Never again may blood of bird
    or beast
Stain with its venomous
    stream a human feast,
To the pure skies in
    accusation steaming.
Avenging poisons shall have
    ceased
To feed disease and fear and
    madness;
The dwellers of the earth
    and air
Shall throng around our steps
    in gladness,
Seeking their food or refuge
    there.
Our toil from thought all
    glorious forms shall cull,
To make this Earth, our
    home, more beautiful;
And Science, and her sister
    Poesy,
Shall clothe in light the fields
    and cities of the free!"*

---

1. This lecture was given by Anna Kingsford on the 24th April 1882, before the Students of Girton College, Cambridge; "And Inscribed to them with Sincere Regard." It

was printed as a pamphlet, a second edition of which was issued in 1884, by the Vegetarian Society (Manchester).

2. "***Scarlet Fever and Butcher's Meat.*** – The rapidly accumulating evidence as to the influence of food in spreading infectious disease has recently received a remarkable addition at the hands of Dr. Robertson, who, in his last annual report on the health of the Penrith Rural District, includes an account of several cases of scarlet fever, which he is strongly inclined to believe were communicated through butcher's meat. In a butcher's family there was an exceedingly mild case of scarlet fever, so mild that no medical man was called in, – the disease, in fact, not being recognised; but the free desquamation of the skin, and the former history of slight fever with sore throat, the leaves no doubt as to the nature of the illness. The occurrence of such a case in a small house, and where no precautions were taken, renders it an easy matter to spread the disease in the manner Dr. Robertson suggests. The number of cases in the neighbourhood continued to increase, notwithstanding all the precautions that were used, in addition to the closure of the schools. The meat is the only means by which Dr. Robertson can imagine the disease was carried in several of the cases; in others, the wanton carelessness of the public, after being fully warned of the danger of having public meetings and private gatherings, was a fruitful cause of its spread. In another village, a large number of cases of scarlet fever occurred, and the health officer has strong reason for suspecting the butcher's meal as a medium by which the infection was spread. The circumstances here were almost identical with those of the first outbreak. The first case was at a butcher's house; it was a slight one, not recognisable by the parents at first; free desquamation took place, and the child was allowed to run all over the premises." – From the ***British Medical Journal***, 15th April 1882.

"*Outbreak of Typhoid in an Infirmary*. – Within the past few days Leicester Infirmary has been the scene of an outbreak of typhoid fever, by which no fewer than ten of the dressers, nurses, and servants have been prostrated, and two others have died. Dr. Buck, the Medical Officer of Health, has instituted an investigation, from which it appears that all the victims had drunk raw milk. As the house-drains appeared to be in good condition, an inquiry was instituted. It was then found that the person who supplied the milk had been affected by similar symptoms, and that the owner of the farm from which it came had also suffered. The farm premises were next inspected. It was ascertained that the well was situated near an overflowing and leaky cesspool, and that it stood near the end of the house-drain. An analysis of three samples was made, and it was shown that the water used for domestic purposes, and with which the milk-cans were washed, was quite unfit for use, being polluted with sewage. It was therefore inferred that the outbreak had arisen from the use of contaminated milk. The patients were, at the last report, progressing favourably."

3. Here follows a passage, beginning with the words "The Perfectionist" and ending with the words "once explicable," similar to that in the first of Anna Kingsford's *Letters on Pure Diet* in **The Food Reform Magazine** (see pp. 65-66, *ante*).
4. **The Revolt of Islam**, Canto V. (li. 5).

4. THE BEST FOOD FOR MAN

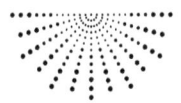

I[1] HAVE said that the French peasantry live much more in accordance with the dictates of Nature than do the English, and that consequently they are, as a rule, far more prosperous and well off. It is a very rare thing indeed for a French peasant to be destitute in his old age, because, although his wages are not nearly so high as in this country, they are much more economically spent, and thrift is looked upon as a cardinal virtue. Hence there is no necessity in France for the unhappy Poor-law system which is the bane of this country, and industrious and frugal householders are not compelled to pay exorbitant taxes for the support of persons who have laid by nothing for themselves. Many of the French peasants have told me how they live. Flesh-meat is so rare on their tables, that, as a rule, it is only eaten two or three times a year, but they take plenty of cheese, coarse bread, vegetable soups and savoury omelettes. On diet like this, with cider to drink, they manage to bring up families of robust, healthy children, to make their homes comfortable, and to lay by savings, sufficient to provide for the old folks when past work. Nor is this the case only in France. It is general all over the greater part of the civilised world. The diet of the Swiss, of the Belgian, the Prussian, the Bavarian, Saxon, Russian, Spanish, Italian, Pomeranian, Norwegian, and Swedish agricultural labourers is almost entirely devoid of flesh-meat. And, as a rule, other things being equal, their vital force and constitution are superior to those of their English brethren, their unstimulating and wholesome food enabling them to work with ease to an advanced age. And here I should like to call attention to a matter of much importance in gauging the extent and quality of vital strength. It should be borne in mind that the proper test of strength is its capacity for endurance. Mere feats of strength are valueless as tests of vital power. The question at issue is not – "How much can a man do in a day?" but "How much can he do in a lifetime?" It is sometimes said by superficial people, – "Beef and beer, will enable you to get through a better day's work than oatmeal or pease pudding." This may be true, generally speaking, because flesh-meat and fermented drinks are both stimulants of the nerves, and under their influence the machinery of the body runs at a faster and more violent rate. But the beef-eater and beer-drinker will probably break down at fifty-five or sixty years of age, because his vitality has been exhausted by forced work in excess of its natural and normal capacity, while the abstainer from these exciting aliments will be a hale man with work in him yet at eighty. It is the old story of the hare and the tortoise.

So then there are three distinct claims established for economy, on the part of the diet without flesh-food: First, it is the most economical as regards the relation between the Land and the People, viz.: cultivated land yielding corn, roots, and vegetables will support a population at least three or four times larger than the same extent of soil laid down in pasture; and this for a two-fold reason, because land under cultivation affords work and wages to a large number of hands, – which must otherwise get employment across the seas, – and because also its produce trebles or quadruples that of land devoted to cattle-grazing.

Secondly a non-flesh diet is the most economical as regards housekeeping. A shilling's worth of oatmeal with fruit and good vegetables will yield as much nourishment and satisfy the appetite better than five shillings' worth of flesh; and if we assume that, on the average, the population of the United Kingdom were to reduce their consumption of animal food by only one pound a week per head, it would give a saving of ten or twelve million pounds sterling a year. A vegetable dietary, to which we may add cheese, milk, butter, and eggs, costs three times less than a mixed dietary of flesh and vegetables.

Thirdly the reformed diet is more economical as regards Human life and strength. Even if you are fortunate enough to escape suffering and disease from some of the horrible disorders to which we have seen flesh-eaters, especially among the poorer classes, are liable, you will probably have to pay with premature infirmity and shortened life the penalty exacted for indulgence in unnatural food. If you burn your candle at both ends you must not expect the material to last so long as it otherwise would.

I may add to these three important economies a fourth, which is worth your serious consideration.

The costliest and the commonest vice in the United Kingdom, especially among the poorer classes, is the vice of drink. And it is the invariable accompaniment of flesh-eating. Strong meats and strong drinks always go together. There is in flesh-food a principle, variously named by medical authorities, which causes a certain irritable condition of the interior coats of the stomach and intestines, and provokes a desire for stimulating drink. This fact is so well known in institutions for the cure of dipsomania, or drunkenness, that in most bad cases abstinence from flesh-foods is enjoined, and in one establishment, unusually successful in its treatment (Dansville, U.S.), no patient entering the hospital is allowed, on any account, during the whole of his residence there, to eat flesh-meat. In fact, we have only to walk down a street in the poorer quarters of a town to see how public-houses or gin palaces abound; and it has many times been pointed out by able observers that the proximity of slaughter-houses, placed, as they invariably are, in the low quarters of a town, incites the inhabitants around to drink to an unusual extent. The frequency of crime as the immediate or proximate result of drinking habits seems to indicate that could we but reach the mainspring of this national curse and arrest its action, we should go far towards arresting altogether the more serious crimes of the country. Anyone who will collect for a week or more the instances appearing at the Police Courts, of what are known as crimes of violence, wife and baby murder, savage assaults and suicide, will see that almost all of them are due to drink. This is an admitted fact; but it is not so generally admitted that the way to the gin palace is through the butcher's shop. Vegetarians never drink to excess. Not all are abstainers on principle from alcohol, many take an occasional glass of wine or beer, but none drink to excess, because their food, being succulent and unstimulating, does not give rise to thirst. What an economy would the adoption of such a diet prove in houses where half the week's earnings now go to buy liquor! Sometime ago a working-man at Manchester made an effective temperance address in the public street. In his hands he held a loaf of bread and a knife. The loaf represented the wages of the working-man. First he cut off a moderate slice. "This," said he, "is what you give to the city government." He then cut off a more generous slice, – "And this," he went on, "is what you give to the general government." Then, with a Vigorous flourish of his carving knife, he cut off three-quarters of the whole loaf. "This," he said, "you give to the brewer and to the public-house." "And this," he concluded, showing the thin slice which remained, "you keep to support yourselves, your families, and to pay the rent."

Now, perhaps some of you, who are not used to vegetarian ways, may be wondering what non-flesh-eaters have for dinner. Well, they have a much larger variety of dishes than eaters of beef, mutton, and pork. But the diet of the vegetarian is a scientific diet, and either knowledge or experience must teach him the nutritive values of foodstuffs, before he can make a wholesome and frugal use of them. All foods contain certain elements necessary to the building up of the material and the renewal of the force of the body, but these elements are contained in very different proportions in various foods. Scientific men have divided the nutritive properties of food into two categories which include respectively: Tissue-forming substances, and Force or Heat-forming substances. They call the first Nitrogenous, and the second, Carbonaceous. Now, both these necessary kinds of food are abundant in the vegetable kingdom, and, proportionately to the weight, there is a great deal more of them to be got out of farinaceous and leguminous matter than out of dead flesh. An adult man in good health, says Dr. Lyon Playfair, requires every day four ounces of nitrogenous or flesh-forming substance, and ten or eleven of carbonaceous or heat and force-giving substance. He can get these elements of nutrition out of bread, oatmeal, pease, cheese, and vegetables at a cost more than less by half that of the butcher's meat necessary to furnish the same amount of nourishment. It is chemically and physiologically demonstrated that no property whatever, beyond that of stimulation, exists in flesh-meat that is not to be found in vegetable food, and that, therefore, it is a terrible error to suppose flesh-meat to be more strengthening than other aliments. It is, in fact, the reverse which is the case, for the quantity of nutriment contained in corn-meal is, for every hundred parts, more than double, sometimes treble – that contained in the same quantity of butcher's meat. The most nutritious and strengthening of all foods are the grains, – the fruit of the cereals, – wheat, oats, barley, rye, rice, maize, and such mealy vegetables as beans, haricots, pease, lentils and their kind. All sorts of fruit are rich in carbo-hydrates, or sugary food, which, according to many medical authorities, is the most necessary of all to the human system. Dr. Playfair puts down the daily proportion of sugary food necessary to an adult man at eighteen ounces – that is more than four times the amount of nitrogenous food requisite. This indispensable item cannot be got out of flesh-meat **at all**, but it is plentiful in table vegetables, such as potatoes, beetroot, tomato, cauliflower, turnips, carrots, parsnips, and so on. The Vegetarian Society has issued a series of excellent little Cookery books, varying in price from half a crown to a penny, giving **recipes** for any number of good cheap meals, without fish, flesh, or fowl. You cannot do better than study these, if you wish to live economically and purely, and to bring healthy children into the world.

Most of the diseases which fill our hospitals are self-induced, having their cause in debauched habits, sometimes aggravated by hereditary malady. Children are born blind, or rickety, or scrofulous, or tuberculous, or idiotic on account of the feeding and drinking habits of their parents. They are bred up under circumstances of incessant vice and misery, and they suck gin with their mother's milk. Hardly weaned, they are given pork and offal for food; their bones give way, their flesh ulcerates, the mothers and the parish doctor together make matters worse by the administration of drugs, and at length the wretched little sufferers, masses of disease and uncleanness, are brought to the hospital. Or, already vitiated in childhood, the average man or woman of the poorer class, ignorant of the laws of health and of the construction of the human body, continues in the way in which his or her early years were bent, and accumulates disease by constant recourse to that which originally caused it, until, at forty or fifty years of age, the pauper ward or the hospital bed receives the unhappy patient, incurably afflicted with some organic complaint. It is simply frightful to the educated mind to hear the confessions of some of these poor bed-ridden creatures. When a student in the hospitals, I was often unable to credit their accounts of the quantities and kinds of strong drinks they had swallowed on a daily average while in work. The question of diet, – what we ought to eat and drink – is the question which underlies everything else and affords the key to the cause of all the accumulation of suffering and moral evil which we meet in poor districts, and especially in cities. Hygiene and morals go hand in hand and are inseparable, just as body and mind make one person, so intimately welded together, that neither good nor harm can be done to the one without affecting the other. This consideration brings me to the most important of all the aspects of flesh-eating, viz., its immoral tendency.

We have seen one of its indirectly immoral results in the fondness it sets up for strong drink, but I am now about to speak of the degrading and barbarous nature of the habit itself, as it affects the national customs, manners, and tone of thought. It needs no very great penetration to see what harm the proximity of slaughter-houses and the loathsome surroundings of the trade must do in the poorer quarters of towns, – the only parts in which these places are to be found. The rich and refined classes shut these things out of sight and hearing, but they are forced upon the poor, and their results are potent for evil. How is it possible to teach poor children the duties of humane treatment of dumb creatures and of tenderness to beasts of burden when their infancy and youth are spent in familiarity with the scenes which surround the slaughter-house, and while they are taught to look upon these institutions and on all they involve as lawful, right, and necessary to man? It is heart-rending to be in the vicinity of the shambles of a large town when its victims are being driven in. Bewildered oxen, footsore, galled, and bruised, sheep with frightened faces, scared at the baying of dogs and the sticks and goads so freely wielded by the roughs who drive them, – little brown-eyed calves, for whose loss the patient mother cows are lowing in the homestead; – all the sad, terrible procession of sacrifice that enters every city at dawn to feed the human multitude that calls itself civilised, – these are the sights upon which the early-rising children of the poor are educated. And a little later in the morning may be heard from within the slaughterhouse the cries of the dying, and the thud of the pole-axe upon the brow of some innocent miserable beast, and the gutters begin to run with blood; and presently the gates of the slaughter-yard open, and out comes a cart or two laden with pailfuls of blood and brains and fresh skins, reeking with the horrible odour of violent death. Are spectacles and sounds like these fit for the eyes and ears of little children, or indeed for any human creature, young or old? It is useless to urge that the Bible justifies the slaughter of animals for food. The Bible seems to sanction a great many practices which modern civilisation and philosophy have unanimously condemned, and which have been made penal offences in all Western codes of law. Such, for instance, are the practices of polygamy and of slavery, which are not only sanctioned in the Bible, but are in some cases positively enjoined. Even murder itself appears to be vindicated in some parts of the Old Testament, as are also many revengeful and cruel acts. No civilised general in these days would dream of conducting warfare as Joshua, as Deborah, as Samuel, or as David conducted it – such deeds as theirs would be justly held to sully the brightest valour; no minister of religion in our times could endure to redden his hands daily with the blood of scores of lambs, doves, and oxen; no average man, woman, or child could be induced to assist in stoning to death an unfortunate "fallen woman," or a lad who had disobeyed his parents or used strong language. Yet these are some of the practices commended and inculcated in the Bible, and justifiable on the same grounds as the practice of flesh-eating.

But the Hebrew Bible is not the only sacred Book in the World. Other "holy Scriptures," known as the Vedas, the Puranas, the Tripitaka, and the Dhammapada, which form the Canon of the religions professed by the largest part of mankind, enjoin abstinence from flesh-food upon all religious persons and extend the command, "Thou shalt not kill," to all creatures, human and animal, which are not noxious and dangerous to the interests of peace and order. In regard to this subject, the Archbishop of Canterbury, at the annual meeting of the Church Missionary Society on 1st May of the present year (1883), said: –

"There are beautiful fruits belonging to the ancient civilisations of the East which we shall work into our Gospel, and our children, ages and generations hence, will wonder how we found the Gospel quite complete without them. Take such a noble thought as the Buddhist thought of the perfect sacredness of Life, how everything that lives, down to the mere animated dust, is a sacred thing. The Buddhist sees the difference between life and everything else that God has made, and it gives to him a tenderness and a sweetness, and a power of union with the creation, which, when we have apprehended it, will enable us to see better and deeper and nobler meanings in St Paul's eighth chapter to the Romans."

These are good words of the Archbishop, and worthy of our serious thoughtfulness. It is not the letter, but the spirit of the Bible which is our true guide. The letter is subject to error, it belongs to the things of time, and has become the stumbling-block of the critics; but the spirit is the true Word of God; it is catholic, vital, and progressive. It is always **with us**, leading us into all truth, as we are able to bear it; but the letter is behind us and behind the age, it is dead, and killeth all who make an idol of it.

It has always seemed to me a strange and horrible anomaly that every one of the great Festivals of the present Christian Church is marked by some wholesale sacrifice of living creatures to our depraved appetites. Christmas, Shrove-tide, Easter, Michaelmas, all are made the occasions of special slaughter. And the season of "peace and good will" is, above all others, selected by common consent as that of universal bloodshed and violence! So soon as "the time draws near the birth of Christ," the streets of city and hamlet everywhere run with blood, and the knife and the pole-axe make havoc among the patient-eyed beasts of the stall, in whose presence, tradition says, the Holy Child made his advent on earth. What a basis is this for Christian civilisation! What associations are these with which to familiarise the minds of our children! How many among the tens of thousands of worshippers in church and chapel throughout the land on Christmas Day give so much as one minute's thought of regret to the incalculable suffering and cruelty caused to our "poor relation," the domestic animals, in order to celebrate the reign of One who is called the "Prince of Peace"? How many think with any shame or sorrow of the human ministers to all this gluttony and selfishness: – of the butchers and slaughter-men passing their lives in scenes of loathsome bloodshed and among unwholesome fumes of death, – of the demoralisation and deterioration of body and mind, of which the perpetration of so much cruelty and savagery must be the inevitable cause?

We trust, – we who live in the Future rather than in the Past or Present, – that the dawn of a better day is about to rise upon our world. Year by year the Spirit of Christ grows mightier and its meaning clearer, as one by one the mists of superstition and misconception melt and drop away from the Holy Name, and we learn that the history of Man is the history of perpetual struggle after the Ideal, of perpetual aspiration after the "more excellent way." This Ideal, this Way, which is also the Truth and the Life, constitute the Christ in man, the ever-living, ever-risen Lord, – to follow whom is to follow "all things lovely, just, pure, and of good report."

It will be seen that the view I take of this question, "What is the Best Food for Man?" involves considerations far transcending the mere physical or economical plane. There is a Best Food for Man which implies a Best mode of Living, a Way into which all paths converge, leading to one celestial goal. This is the Way of Paradise, which is, equally, the Way of the Cross, because it is the will of God, and, therefore, the law of the universe, that no perfection is possible in anything but by means of self-denial and self-conquest. The ordinary flesh-eater, if he be a man of any perception, is always fain to acknowledge, on being pressed, that there is something in the usual mode of feeding which clashes with his finer sense of what ought to be. He would rather not talk about the slaughter-house, he feels that the whole subject is, somehow, unsavoury, and more or less frankly admits that he cannot associate the idea of slaughter with what are called "Utopian" theories of existence. But, in most cases, he is not ready to sacrifice the least of his appetites to his conscience. He likes the taste of flesh-meat, he will tell you, and does not wish to deprive himself of the pleasure it gives him. It is the custom of Society to eat it, and he has no desire to make himself conspicuous by refusing to partake of the dishes set before him by his friends. Such an attitude of mind, of course, can only be dealt with effectually by an effort of will on the part of the individual himself. The excuses thus formulated are precisely those with which every transgressor of every moral law turns to bay on the man who seeks to reform or convict him. The reason of such a man may be amply convinced that flesh-eating is neither scientific nor civilised, and yet he lacks the courage to carry these convictions into practice. No logic is able to influence a person of this kind. His affair is with his Conscience rather than with his reason.

But sometimes we meet opponents who tell us that the plea for purer and more merciful living rests on mere "sentiment." Beasts kill one another, they say, therefore man may kill beasts. And if he did not so kill them, they would so increase in numbers that he himself would become their prey. Let us examine the value of these arguments. It is no shame or reproach to us that a large part of our doctrine rests upon the basis of the sentiments. It must necessarily be so if the doctrine be really a scientific and reasonable doctrine, because God and Nature are not at strife but in harmony, and that mode of living which is best fitted for our bodies and most helpful to the development of our minds is, of course, most in harmony with our moral nature. Nature has not made the consumption of flesh necessary or suitable to the human organism, and the bodily needs of man are not, therefore, in continual antagonism to his reason and to his spiritual instincts. Were it otherwise, we should be forced to admit the tendencies of civilisation and of morality to be at war with the dictates imposed by natural law. And it is precisely the power to recognise and exercise the sentiments which makes man to differ from the beasts. The glory of humanity does not lie in its physical form, for, from time immemorial, the world has seen brutes in human shape, with whose ferocity, malignity, and lust no lower animal could compare. Nor does it lie in sagacity, or perfection of method in mechanical contrivance, – the basis of all we call Intellect; for on this ground, the mere bee, the ant, the beaver, the bird, the fox, the dog, compete with and even surpass us, as may easily be ascertained by any observer of nature. Nor does man's superiority rest on his physical strength, for what is his muscular force compared with that of the elephant, the rhinoceros, or any of the terrible beasts of jungle, forest, and plain? It is none of these things that makes man; but it *is* the possession of moral reason, the conception, practice and veneration of Truth, Love, Mercy, Justice, Self-denial, Honour, Charity. And these are the sentiments. And our system of living is pre-eminently a sentimental system, founded in the nature of Humanity, and made for true Men.

The rule which applies, therefore, to the lower

animals, – our brothers in all but in the development of spiritual faculties, – is no rule for us, and cannot be twisted into a criterion for our conduct, or an apology for our cruelties. If we are to justify ourselves in killing and eating them because some of the fiercer races among them kill and eat one another, we might, by the same logic, descend to their plane in respect of all other practices attractive to low-minded and vicious men, and revert to polygamy, disregard of personal rights, and still worse manners. For if certain animals see no harm in bloodshed, neither do they see harm in theft, rapine, and seduction.

As for the objection that unless we ate our animal brethren, they would eat us, nothing can be more ill-considered or pointless. One would suppose the objector to be under the impression that cattle, sheep, and other market animals grow wild like trees or grass, instead of being the objects of an elaborate system of forcing, breeding, rearing, buying, and selling. It would be quite as logical to fear being devoured by our unused potatoes and turnips as to dread being eaten up by our herbivorous animals! For these creatures are exactly in the position of the edible crops we plant annually for our use, and if they were not artificially bred, they would rapidly diminish in numbers, change their character, and return to the orderly balance of Nature. The fact is that the force of our objector's argument is all the other way, and that it is precisely to the flesh-eating habits of our present population that we owe a very real danger of being eaten up by flocks and herds. For in order to meet the exorbitant demand for animal food and for field sports, thousands of English men and women are annually compelled to give place to cattle and to sheep runs; land which would support scores of families with corn and crops is laid waste for pasture, for cover, for warrens, for preserves, for deer-forests; and the peasantry and the agriculturists, eaten out of house and home by beasts, are forced to congregate in overstocked towns, whose streets are hideous with the plague of drink-shops, slaughter-yards, and meat-markets; or else to quit their native shores and seek a new world far off beyond the seas.

Under our present regimen, the beasts of fold and of cover usurp the people's rights, and with this usurpation come the accompanying evils of poverty, dirt, squalor, drink, crime, the enforced exile of field labourers, and the consequent surplus of a helpless female population of a million souls, condemned thus, inevitably, to a loveless and lonely life, or to the alternative of misfortune and shame.

Is it too much to ask of the human race that it should consent to restore the world to the dominion of natural law and order; – that it should sacrifice the luxury and sensuality of the Few to the peace and joy of the Many, and that it should learn to be wise, clean, pure, thrifty, and virtuous?

Is it too much to ask the suppression of an organised system of carnage, involving a foul and unhealthy traffic, disgusting occupations, depraving spectacles, and gross barbarity? – To plead for the restoration of Beauty in the morals of the people, in the surroundings of daily life, in the haunts and homes of the poor; in the sports and at the banquets of the rich? Surely not, for alike from the scientific, the hygienic, the aesthetic, and the spiritual point of view, the Best Food for Man is that which does no violence to his nature, physical or moral, and which involves none to other creatures at his hand. For this we are Men, that alone of all Nature's children we should be able to understand the secret of her manifold transmutations, and the goal of her striving; for this we are Men, that we may be able to confirm her inspiration by our Reason, and that, standing open-eyed and face to face with our nursing mother, we may know what the best of our younger brothers only dimly feel, and grasp with strong, mature, responsible sense knowledges that are with them but instincts, and virtues which their undeveloped minds reflect as inborn impulse merely. Thus may Man endorse the work of God, becoming its exponent and interpreter while others remain its objects, and realise upon a higher and spiritual plane the beautiful intentions of the Divine Mind in the world of natural forms and evolutions. And the more he himself becomes uplifted towards that Mind, the more also will he love and pity and long for harmony with all innocent incarnations of life in the great universe of Being.

---

1. This article was written by Anna Kingsford, and was published (in two parts) in the **Theosophist** of February and of March 1884.

5. THE PHYSIOLOGY OF VEGETARIANISM

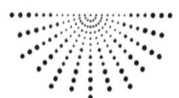

I[1] SHALL put before you, principally, the scientific aspects of the question. First, I will speak of the misunderstanding under which we Vegetarians lie. Only two days ago I took up a popular society paper in which Vegetarians were spoken of as "poor, crazy creatures flying in the face of nature." Another writer spoke of us, in the ***Times***, as "poor weaklings." I don't think that phrase exactly applicable to us or our history, either past, present, or future as Vegetarians. As there is a great deal of misapprehension about, let me point out a few facts about Vegetarianism scientifically considered. Some have the idea that we would send out men to graze like Nebuchadnezzar. They never seem to have heard of the class of animals called "frugivorous." They can never have read Huxley, or the works of the great anatomists and physiologists. They have never followed the arguments on the doctrine of evolution. I won't say if I am an evolutionist or not. On one point there is no doubt whatever: if we study the anatomy of man, we find it is just the same as that of the higher apes; both are anatomically and physiologically the same. This is a little against our pride, perhaps, to think that we only belong to the family of apes; but I am not speaking of their moral qualities. If you go into a dissecting room and see an ape on one table and a human creature on another, you have a great deal of difficulty in seeing the difference between them, especially if the skin has been stripped off. The teeth of man are precisely the same as the teeth of the ape. We hear a great deal from people, who don't understand it, about the canine teeth. These, they say, are flesh-tearing teeth. They are nothing of the sort. The cuspid teeth of the ape are for the purpose of defence and of cracking nuts, and certainly under no circumstances for eating beefsteaks or mutton chops. A grown man has thirty-two teeth, if he has them all, wisdom teeth included. There are apes of the Old World, and apes of the New. The apes of the Old World have thirty-two teeth also. The teeth of the ape are exactly the same as those of man, in form and method of growth. Will anyone say that the ape is carnivorous. If you go to any of our great museums or menageries, here or abroad, you will find the rations of the apes are apples, bread, and so forth. The keepers perfectly well recognise that the ape is not a carnivorous animal. I don't want to dwell too long upon this question of anatomy, or I could prove that in the formation of the mouth, the stomach, and the intestinal canal, man is exactly the same as an ape. Among the great writers on anatomy or physiology, you find no difference of opinion. Thus the food of man is fixed by science – and science is a very hard thing to argue against. Man is formed to eat the fruits of the earth, and not to eat flesh. If man has adapted himself to eat flesh, it is by custom, not by nature. With regard to the economical aspect of the question, we are told Vegetarians cannot be strong; it is impossible to have force unless you eat meat. Let us look at the question scientifically. The food needed by the body can be divided into two great classes – nitrogenous and carbonaceous. If you try experiments upon man, you will find that these two great classes answer two great purposes in the economy of the human body. The nitrogenous food goes to form muscle and tissue; the carbonaceous gives heat and force. It has been calculated that the amount of nitrogenous and carbonaceous matter we require – taken according to the proportions of Dr. Pavy, Dr. Edward Smith, and others – is of nitrogenous four to five ounces, and of carbonaceous fifteen to twenty-two ounces daily. The carbons are divided into two groups, the hydro-carbons and the carbo-hydrates; these are hard names. The hydro-carbons are all oils and fats; the carbo-hydrates are all starches and sugars. According to Dr. Playfair, the starches and sugars are necessary in the proportion of seventeen to eighteen ounces every day. With one single exception, these are obtained from the vegetable kingdom. It is necessary that we should absorb a certain quantity of sugar; there is no sugar to be found, except in milk, out of the vegetable kingdom. We will glance at the approximate value of these foods, and see how very much richer the vegetable kingdom is. We hear it said: "If you want to build up muscle and tissue and so on, you must go to the animal kingdom for it. If you wish to be strong you must consume nitrogenous matter contained in flesh-meat." Now, pork and ham contain 8 %, lean beef and mutton 18 % of nitrogenous matter; flesh-meats thus contain from 8 to 18 %. If you get your nitrogen from the vegetable kingdom, you will find it much cheaper. You get from 25 to 30 % of nitrogenous matter out of lentils, pease, beans, and all kinds of cereals. With regard to the carbonaceous foods, we get all we need from the vegetable kingdom. And the oils too are far more cleanly when obtained from the vegetable than from the animal kingdom. This is clear to the meanest capacity, and I do not dwell upon the point. Again, animals are liable to many diseases. All the worm diseases proceed from eating animal food, and the poor get the worst kinds of meat; that is, they are obliged to get the intestines, the lights and liver, precisely those parts where the germs of disease abound. These germs of disease are not to be seen by the naked eye, but as soon as they get into the human frame they develop slowly and surely. In the intestinal canal, perhaps, there is a tiny speck, hardly to be seen by the aid of the microscope. Yet this may develop into a worm four or five feet long. Nor is that the only animal disease. Another disease, well known to butchers, is "pearl" disease, which is a form of tubercular disease. We heard the other day of butcher's meat being 80 to 90 % diseased. We even can give for this the authority of Dr. Alfred Carpenter, speaking before the Medical Congress of 1881; so we may take it for granted it is true, yet it seems almost incredible, that from 80 to 90 % of butcher's meat should be unfit for food. Put it down at a lower figure, and you may say that 60 to 70 % is diseased. This is frightful when you come to think of it. From the worm diseases the vegetable kingdom is absolutely free. Men may, of course, get unsound vegetables, but they are easily seen to be not good, and we do not eat them. Meat, however, deceives us; it may look perfectly well, and we may not be aware of disease in it, but it may contain the very germs I mentioned just now. Now, about one of the "strong" arguments our opponents adduce. They say if we did not kill animals we should have our fields and back gardens swarming with cattle! It is amusing that people do not stop for a moment to see what this means. Is it not perfectly well known that we breed animals to kill? They say if we do not destroy the bullocks and other animals we shall have sheep and oxen running all about the streets. We should be eaten out of house and home by cows. We should soon see if they were indigenous to this country, were all the people Vegetarians. The fact is that the land which ought to be the people's is given to the beasts. In this England of ours we want to have the cottagers on their own land. We want to have this land of England cultivated as a garden, and not left for sheep to wander over and for game deer to run wild in. We want to prevent men being sent out of the country as they are now. Now, many of the best and ablest of the people cannot find work, so they cross the seas and leave behind them a surplus of women, a mass of terrible distress and awful sin and misery. We want to give the land back to the people, that they may live in an economical and happy manner; that when old they may live on their savings by their own firesides. You know, perhaps, in foreign countries, especially in France, there are no workhouses. They live there in a very economical manner, in order to keep their homes together, the result being that whole families gather together round one fireside, and in one cottage, instead of being separated as in England, where we send old people to the workhouse, and our sons over the sea to find bread. Instead of pressing large numbers into degrading occupations, now necessitated by the requirements of the people, were we to be Vegetarians, at once these would be set free. How much more happily they could live on vegetable produce! It is lamentable that the poor have the idea that no food is good except meat. A friend of mine used to give the poor in his neighbourhood vegetable soup, and they gladly received it at first; but as soon as they found there was no "stock" in the soup they would not have it. This is a very common idea. Who should be blamed for it? We have the doctors to blame. In the hospitals again and again we hear the words, "You must take flesh-meat," or, "You know you must get some port wine," and that sort of thing. Well, my own experience is this – I cured myself of tubercular consumption by living on vegetable food. A doctor told me I had not six months to live. What was I to do? I was to eat **raw meat** and drink port wine.

Well, I went into the country and ate porridge and fruit, and appear to-day on this platform! Then, again, there is the Leather Question. I was determined that on this point I would not have my boots thrown at my head as a reproach; so I went about London to find a man who would make boots without leather, and I found him, and have the boots on this evening. The argument about leather then is answered, for soles, uppers, and everything else are made without it. Two years ago I climbed the hills of Switzerland in boots made without leather. I have pretty well solved this question, then. When there comes a demand for boots made without leather, you will be able to get them. I am afraid I have over-talked my time now. I had a great many things to say, but I am afraid I shall forget them. There is much to say with regard to the history of Vegetarianism. There have been a great many very illustrious names connected with Vegetarianism: men of such calibre as Gautama Buddha, whose life has been given to the world in that beautiful poem, **The Light of Asia**, which is now issued as cheap as possible – at one shilling. You should read that work and the teaching of Edwin Arnold, and if that does not convert you to Vegetarianism, nothing will; it is full of the most beautiful language and most pathetic sentiment possible to imagine. You will find that a book to smile over, and a book to weep over. It is the sort of literature I should like to see widely disseminated in London. I could point to such men as Pythagoras, as Seneca the friend of St Paul, and to a whole army of Vegetarian saints – in the Church and out of it; to Shelley, the king of poets, to whose beautiful poem, **Queen Mab**, there is appended a long note in the form of an "*Essay on Flesh-eating*." Plutarch, too, is with us, and all the greatest teachers and philosophers in the world. It does not seem much as if we are "poor weaklings." Physically, too, the gorilla, which is a Vegetarian, is one of the strongest animals. Du Chaillu tells us how once he was frightened by a gorilla, and dropped his gun, which that animal took up and snapped in two as though it had been a hazel twig! Yet this gorilla was fed on nuts and fruits. Well, the hardest work of the world in our cities, and in our battle-fields, and in our wheat-fields too, is done by animals which, side by side with us, build our towns and cultivate our lands, and are Vegetarians. So, from a physical point of view, we repudiate the epithet of "poor weaklings." And we do so as regards intellect also. With regard to the moral point of view, we have a tower of strength, and can easily prove we are not "poor weaklings." I think on every point we can prove our strength, and, let me say it with all modesty, our superiority also. We are superior to animals of prey, and we rise above them. We don't want to drag ourselves down to the level of the tiger, but we rather rise above it. Our motto is "Upwards and onwards!" We should strive to teach men to live simply and purely, and we should reduce our own wants as much as we can. We should assimilate ourselves more and more to the teaching of those men who have been pioneers of the cause. Let us adopt the teaching of Pythagoras – "Learn to love that which is right, and custom will make it pleasant and delightful." I will close my remarks by quoting two verses of a little poem [2] of Goldsmith, which perhaps you have heard. They appear to place our doctrine in a beautiful light, so I don't think I can do better than quote them to you. They are very simple, yet they are very expressive. They are:

> *"No flocks that range the valley free*
> *To slaughter I condemn;*
> *Taught by the Power that pities me,*
> *I learn to pity them.*
>
> *But from the mountain's grassy side*
> *A guiltless feast I bring;*
> *A scrip with fruit and corn supplied,*
> *And water from the spring."*

---

1. From the Report of the Address given by Anna Kingsford on 12th January 1885 at Exeter Hall, London, at the close of the International Health Exhibition, under the auspices of the Manchester Vegetarian Society. It is one of many addresses that were, on that occasion, given by prominent vegetarians; it is taken from the Report of the Exeter Hall Meeting that was issued by the above-mentioned society.
2. In ***The Vicar of Wakefield***.

6. HISTORICAL ASPECT OF FOOD REFORM

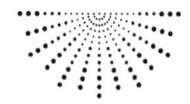

IT[1] has been allotted to me to speak of the historical development of this form of diet, and I think a reference to evolution quite necessary in this connection, for one can hardly take up the history of man at any given period without referring it back to the sources from which he sprang. For we must look upon the human race, not as a thing apart from the rest of creation, but as being in brotherhood and solidarity with the whole of those living forms with which we are surrounded. From the scientific point of view we all arise out of differentiation from one common stock; but the one point I wish to dwell upon is that there has been throughout that evolution a steady heading towards the best, a steady "stream of tendency which makes for righteousness"; and we see that evolution has been accomplished by the gathering up into the complex nervous structure, and especially into the large ganglion of the brain, of all the best that nature can give. That is to say, that it is by the elaboration of the nervous structure, and especially of the brain, that man has become man. I wish in connection with this subject to point out to you that man sprang immediately from the frugivorous group. It is a fact of great significance, that man became man as a fruit-eater, and not as a carnivorous animal, for it shows that the carnivora were incapable of producing man, and that the frugivorous group alone were capable of the necessary elaboration and perfection of the intellectual nature. The recognition of this fact must be an enormous gain to food reform. It is sometimes said to me, when I dwell on the anatomy and physiology of man in connection with this question, that he could just as well have sprung out of the races of the tiger or the lion or the jackal. But I say no; the very fact that he did not, proves those races incapable of such evolution. When you know that all the great anatomists have agreed to place the primates – the great anthropoid apes – at the head of the whole family of natural evolution, and have classed them according to the structural evolution of the nervous system, you see that we may claim for this frugivorous group the ascendancy and priority over all the rest. And not only is it true in connection with the ape; it is also true in connection with all the first races of man.

I do not care whether you take up your Ovid or your Hesiod or your Bible, you will find always the same tale. You will find that in the Golden Age (if you turn to your Ovid) men lived upon the fruits of the earth and upon such natural gifts as kind nature bestowed on them, "nor stained their lips with blood." So, if you turn to the first chapter of Genesis you will find the command was to "eat the fruits of the earth."

Whether you take the popular religious point of view, the scientific point of view, or the poetic point of view, you always come to the same thing; all have their starting-point in the frugivorous dispensation; and from it have sprung all the great nations which gave us the laws, the sciences, and arts which the world has since elaborated. In Sharpe's **History of Egypt** it is stated that the law-givers of primitive Egypt prohibited the use of flesh; and I hardly need remind you that it is from Egypt that the Western world has received all the best that it now has of science and of knowledge. When we think of the builders of the pyramids, the mighty givers of the philosophy of the past – when we dwell upon the profound thoughts of those great men – when we remember the arts and sciences they have left behind, we perceive what we owe to that past – that past which lives so finely, so subtilly, and so splendidly in the pages of history.

Turn again to the East. They say Pythagoras, the Sage of Samos, learned all his knowledge in the East – but this point, of course, we are not discussing – however, this fact remains, that all the great tribes of India are frugivorous in their habits, and when we study the laws of the Brahmins, we find them divided into several sects or classes – castes, as they are called. The three first castes, the highest of course, are precluded from the use of animal meat – in fact the use of animal meat is associated in the minds of these Eastern people with the idea of pollution, and they allow it only therefore to the lowest class, an idea exactly opposite to that to which we are accustomed in the West. I conversed with a Brahmin some years ago, a Brahmin who had broken his caste by crossing the sea. On learning what the custom of this country was he resolved before leaving his native country to accustom himself, in silence and darkness, to the degrading habit of eating flesh-meat. He was forced to eat it at night with the door shut for fear of his people coming upon him and discovering his apostasy. There was, however, one man in the house where he resided who was obliged to know of his habits. This one man was his servant, a member of the lowest class, who used to supply his master with the meat, so that he might habituate himself to a diet which he understood to be common in the country which he was about to visit. After a time the Brahmin noticed that various things about his house were stolen, valuables disappeared; he suspected this man who waited upon him, and he charged him with theft, and said to him: "I will bring you before the magistrate and accuse you of robbing me." Then the servant turned upon him at once, and said: "You dare not; for if you do I will bring against you a charge of the horrible crime of which you are guilty in the silence of the night, and the revelation of which would degrade you from your caste." And so the Brahmin was forced to hold his peace. You may gather from this something of the ingrained idea prevalent in the East of the pollution which a man undergoes by breaking his caste and eating flesh. I merely narrate this little story to show you how strongly this idea in the matter of caste is held among the Brahmins and Buddhists. Gautama Buddha (than whom I believe there never lived in the world more gentle, more admirable, or more holy being) taught this doctrine to his disciples as the most precious and integral part of his teaching. He laid it down as a rule that no man should take the life of any living creature, and the whole tendency of the teachings of Buddha and of the Buddhist religion lies in this direction. I agree entirely with the Archbishop of Canterbury when he said, some time ago, that we ought to blend the teachings of the Gospel with the almost divine evangel of Gautama Buddha, and that we ought to take all that it has of good and incorporate it with ours. If you want to understand something of the religious life of the East you should read the beautiful poem of Edwin Arnold, The Light of Asia, and learn what nobleness, what grandeur there is in the heart of man when he lives aright, as men should live, and becomes that which he is intended to be by nature. Then you will learn how splendid, how sublime, how beautiful, is the philosophy to which he can reach. I think that here, in the West, we shall do well to study the doctrines of Gautama Buddha and of the Buddhist religion. I am always struck with the idea that all the highest, the purest, the subtlest, the most deep-reaching philosophy which the world holds has come to us from the vegetarian races. Not merely is that the case in regard to the Buddhists, but in regard also to the great Egyptian teacher, Hermes Trismegistos, who held the same doctrines. And the whole of the greatest and purest thoughts that have come to us along the channel of time have been filtered down to us, it appears, through these great races.

That is the case, it seems to me, with **thought**. The question that we now have to face is, "Is it the case with physical force?" It has been said: it is all very well for philosophers to live on a vegetarian diet, but when you come to fighting, you must eat flesh as do the warriors of the West, who distinguish themselves by conquest, while the East is distinguished by thought. All the races which – I have been vegetarian, it is said, have been contemplative, philosophic, and meditative races. Those which have been fighting races have been eaters of animal food. Well, that is an intricate question, and I am not quite sure that even if we so decide it we should be wholly in the right, for I remember that the most splendid heroes that the world has ever seen, the Spartans, under Leonidas, who held the Pass of Thermopylae, were livers on barley bread, oatcake, and oil. The heroes of Salamis and of Marathon were well-nigh all vegetarians; so also were the Persians, under Cyrus. When I consider this, I am inclined to think that all the true heroism of the world may fairly be gathered from among the flower of the vegetarian races. Remember, that to be a hero is one thing, and to have an itch and fever for war is another. It is one thing to make a stand with the Spartans and with Gordon, and it is another to long to fly at the throats of our neighbours and deluge the world in blood. He who can stand face to face with his foe calmly, with courage and without flinching, is a hero; but to desire to kill for the sake of conquest, to decimate a country for the passion of war, is an outrage upon human nature.

I think that as long as men live upon the food of the tiger they will have the tiger's nature; but if they adopt the food of the Golden Age, – the food of Eden, I care not which you call it, – they will have the nature of Paradise. If the world is to be redeemed we must get back to that beautiful time which is celebrated by all the poets; which haunts evermore the dreams of the seers; of which Shelley sang – Shelley, the king of poets; – of which all the truest, sublimest, and purest souls of the world have had the divine and beatific vision. Let me cite to you those beautiful and prophetic lines in **The Revolt of Islam**, which foretell this Paradise regained.

[Here the lecturer recited the passage from **The Revolt of Islam** which is to be found at the conclusion of her *Lecture on Food*.]

---

1. Reprinted from a Report, published in **The Food Reform Magazine** (No. I. vol v., July-September 1885, p. 16), of an Address given by Anna Kingsford on Tuesday, 26th May 1855, at Exeter Hall, under the auspices of the National Food Reform Society.

7. SOME ASPECTS OF THE VEGETARIAN QUESTION

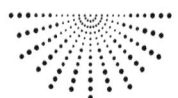

IT[1] appears to me that we may justly regard the century in which we live as **par excellence** the age of Reform and of Criticism. The work of our day seems to be almost exclusively that of applying tests to the discoveries and theories of the past. The civilised world has outgrown its childhood, and consents no longer to take things upon trust. With nations, as with individuals, the enthusiastic faith and credulity of youth yields, in process of time, to the sober reason of maturity. The mind, whether single or aggregate, reviews, with the searching eye of a critic, the opinions it has hitherto entertained, subjects them, one by one, to the test of logic, and retains only such as are sufficiently well-founded to stand the crucial examination unimpaired.

Thus, at the present era of our national history, we are dealing with our old beliefs, and by degrees are putting away our childish things. We are not now satisfied to pursue a certain course of life, or to hold by certain modes of faith, merely because that was the life and this the faith which contented our ancestors. We are asking the meaning and purpose of our existence, and inquiring why such and such things are to be done, and what is our warranty for doing them.

In this manner I account for the fact that the nineteenth century is so fruitful in critics and in censorship. Nothing can be said or done in these days without attracting comment. Everyone who stands forward to advocate any particular cause or opinion is asked why he supports it; nor is it enough for him to reply that the duty of so doing attaches to his hereditary faith or family history. Such an answer would have suited the times that are past very fairly, but the people of to-day want personal convictions which shall bear with impunity the broad light of Reason.

This keen and searching fire of criticism which burns around us may well be likened to the famous cauldron of the enchantress Medea. Into it is put the old worn-out body of the world's past creeds and theories, inert, decrepit, powerless to touch any longer the minds and hearts of the people. But out of the purifying furnace springs the aspiration of the new age, vigorous and strong, full of life and youth and purpose. So it comes about that the popular movements of our time are the result, as a rule, of criticism applied to past ideas. Of late, people have dared to ask why, in old times, wives and daughters were subjected by their male relatives, and practically denied the dignity of humanity. As a result of this inquiry we have the agitation for women's rights. Other people, again, have questioned the sense and propriety of the flesh-eating habits which have prevailed so generally hitherto in European countries, and by consequence the Vegetarian Society rises into being. "Reform" is the cry of our day. With us the inquiry to be made is not "What did our fathers think?" or "What have been the belief and practice of the past?" but more reasonably, "What should *we* think?" "What should be the belief and practice of the ***future***?" The consideration of that which ought to be is now of more importance to us than the consideration of that which has been. It is our duty and our desire to progress beyond our ancestors, not to imitate them. Intellect is ever on the march; the spirit of man is never contented with the possessions of a bygone age; his nature and the law of his being compel him to a continual striving after the highest and the best – that is, the Divine.

And for those who know and estimate the absolute dependence of Mind upon Matter, the Vegetarian movement will assume a vast importance and significance among the progressive theories of the age. We *are* that which we eat; our food is converted into our blood, our blood nourishes our brains, our brains are the *foci* and centres of our thoughts. In the old and beautiful story of the Fall of Man, we find the entire moral and spiritual condition of the individual independent on his choice of food, and a wrong selection in this respect immediately followed by the most dismal results to his soul. It is the same with each of us today. Our whole mental *status* rests upon our bodily condition. If we feed purely and wisely, we shall be pure and wise in spirit. If, on the contrary, we accustom ourselves to gross diet, and mould our appetites to seek and to love food which is obtained at the expense of suffering and death to other sentient creatures, we shall assuredly develop in our souls the sensuality and the cruel tastes of the men of past times. Shall we not, then, place the spiritual progress of our race foremost in the catalogue of our necessities – foremost in our personal aspirations? Shall we not, all of us, combine to sacrifice every consideration of luxury to the higher claims of the soul?

And, again, do we not find, as a matter of fact, that the more earnest and the more advanced a man is in the study and practice of wisdom, the simpler and the more frugal become his habits of diet? Cast your eye back on the biographical records of former times, whether biblical or secular, and you will find that the prophets, the seers, the miracle-workers, the saints, the students, the teachers, the philosophers whose great names make the glory of the Past, were men of exceeding temperance, often ascetics in regard to appetite.

Some persons will tell you that the Divine Founder of the Christian Church was a flesh-eater. The utmost they can show from gospel narrative is that He ate fish, and the obvious inference from several passages is against the supposition that He partook of meat in any grosser form. When hungry in the wilderness, it was with the suggestion of **bread**, and not of flesh, that the demon attempted to beguile His pure desires; when famished with long abstinence and travel, it was with the fruit of the fig-tree that He sought to satisfy His appetite.

But the closing act of His life was one of such deep significance and interest to Vegetarians that I cannot avoid noticing it here. Surely it is at least remarkable that the memorial and type of His mission to the world should have been bequeathed under the emblems of unleavened bread and wine mingled with water. We know that the Jews were accustomed to celebrate the Passover by eating the flesh of a lamb, and this lamb has always been regarded as the type of the Messiah. It might, therefore, have been naturally expected that this same Messiah, celebrating this identical paschal feast, would have chosen the lamb before Him on the table as the type of Himself in time to come, and thus have perpetuated the use of the ancient symbol in the Church He was about to institute. But instead, we find Him consecrating a cake of unfermented meal as his sacramental representative. But instead of this innocent victim, Jesus of Nazareth lays His hand upon a loaf of unleavened grain, and on a cup of unfermented wine, and these He gives to His apostles as the regenerating and bloodless food of the future Church – His legacy to the new-born brotherhood – fittest token and symbol of the gentle morality He advocated, and of the pure and simple aspirations He taught. "This," says He, "is My Body, and this My Blood. These are the untainted elements from whence I draw my perfect Being, my wondrous power and vitality. This is the mysterious meat of which ye knew not; these the aliments on which ye also ought to support your lives. Henceforward eat and drink these in memory of your Master." Thus His last act is to restore to the world a pure dietary, and, dismissing the barbarisms of the past, to assure His disciples that the age of slain victims and of paschal lambs should yield in the wiser hereafter to a more spiritual dispensation. "Whoso eateth this bread and drinketh of this cup for his sustenance shall never see death." There is, rightly, a far more literal meaning in these words of Christ's than theologians are apt to fancy.

Passing from religious to economical considerations, we may notice, first, a very general objection raised with regard to Vegetarianism which we may represent by the query: "What will become of *us* if we do not kill and eat other creatures? Shall we not be ourselves eaten by them?" In the first place I reply: "The animals at present used for human food are artificially bred. Cease to breed them." And in the second place I would observe that there are many creatures which are not used for food which, nevertheless, do not increase to any appreciable, still less to any injurious, extent. Do we think we run any risk of being devoured by badgers, beavers, squirrels, dogs, weasels, hedgehogs, cats, or horses? Or of being pecked to death by robins, wrens, or titmice? Have we not even great difficulty in obtaining horses and other beasts of burden at reasonable prices, although these creatures are never killed for food, save by a few fanatics in Paris? It seems, indeed, that nature is so regulated as to prevent the undue multiplication of any one kind of animal, and that only a fixed and limited number of each species is permitted to exist.

Again, it is not in the least probable that the whole world, or even the members of one nation, or the population of one city, will be converted to Vegetarianism simultaneously. The adoption of a purer system of diet will be a gradual process among us. Therefore, those creatures which are now reared artificially will have ample time to decrease gradually in number as the demand for their flesh gradually lessens and ceases. Most of these animals too, let us recollect, are not indigenous to our climate, but have been at a remote period imported from distant parts of the globe: the ox probably from Oriental countries, the sheep from Africa. That stupidity and docility of manner which we must all have noticed as peculiar to these beasts, and which is frequently remarked upon as a proof that they were created to be our prey, result from the circumstances of their unnatural and domesticated state, and is by no means characteristic of their tribe. Every art which tends to make the poor cow and sheep more helpless and useless to themselves has been adopted by man; and if we are to look for these creatures in their natural condition, we must seek them in the wilds of Tartary, or in the deserts of Africa. Among the captive descendants of the wild kine there have been so many changes wrought by civilisation as strangely to disguise their true nature. Those enfeebled and idolent animals which we see in our fields and streets are a degenerate race, trained by the hand of man, and propagated merely to pamper his vitiated appetites. Nature shows nothing so stupid, so inert, so defenceless.

Stand awhile in any one of our pasture-meadows and observe the sheep. He is a large mass of flesh, supported on four small straight legs, ill-fitted for carrying such a burden. His movements are awkward, he is easily fatigued, and frequently sinks under the weight of his own corpulence. And, in proportion as these marks of human transformation become more numerous and observable, the creature becomes more helpless and stupid. Oxen and sheep which batten upon very fertile lands become fat and entirely feeble, those that lack horns being the most dull and heavy, while those whose fleeces are longest and finest are most subject to disease. In short, whatever changes have been wrought upon these unfortunate brutes by man, are entirely calculated for imagined human advantage and not for that of the creatures themselves. It would require a succession of ages to restore the ox or the sheep to its primitive condition of strength and activity so as to match in point of perfection its compeers of wild or forest.

Sometimes, again, we are told by our opponents that if the whole nation, or any considerable portion of it, were to become Vegetarian, we should not, in our latitude, be able to produce fruits and vegetables in sufficient quantity to meet the demand for food. But imagine all the miles of English pasture and sheep-runs converted into orchards, gardens, and grain fields; imagine the pigstyes, cattle sheds, and pens giving place to fragrant vineyards and fruit-houses! Will anyone be hardy enough to say we should not then have enough to eat and to spare?

Mr. W.R. Greg, in a paper upon population and the prospects of the world in view of the ever-rapidly increasing tide of human life on the earth, observes: "There is one mode in which the amount of human life sustainable on a given area, and therefore throughout the chief portion of the habitable globe, may be almost indefinitely increased, *i.e.* by a substitution of vegetable for animal food. A given acreage of wheat will feed at least ten times as many men as the same acreage employed in growing mutton. It is usually calculated that the consumption of wheat by an adult is about one quarter per annum, and we know that good land produces four quarters. But let us assume that a man living on grain would require two quarters a year; still one acre would support two men. But a man living on meat would need three pounds a day, and it is considered a liberal calculation if an acre spent in grazing sheep and cattle will yield in beef or mutton more than fifty pounds on an average – the best farmer in Norfolk having averaged ninety pounds; but a great majority of farms in Great Britain only reach twenty pounds. On these data, it would require twenty-two acres of pasture-land to sustain one adult person living on meat. It is obvious that, in view of the adoption of vegetable diet, there lies the indication of a vast possible increase in the population sustainable on a given area."

Once more: there is a favourite argument

brought against us on the score of the human teeth. People like to assume that they have carnivorous teeth – the teeth of the lion, the wolf, or the tiger. Well, if our opponents have such teeth, it is because they have developed them by habit through successive generations, just as many other abnormal characteristics of body have been developed in all manner of creatures by means of long-continued custom.

It really happens, however, that the human cuspids (or canine teeth, as they are erroneously called) do not bear the slightest resemblance to those of the carnivorous animals, and it is on the shape and formation of these cuspids that the whole argument of the advocates of flesh-eating depends. In the human jaw there is no space between the opposite teeth for receiving the cuspids, as in the jaws of all carnivorous animals. And in the jaws of the horse, camel, and other individuals of the herbivorous tribes, the canines are considerably longer in proportion to the other teeth than they are in the human jaw; therefore, these creatures must be held, if we are to be logical in our deductions, far more carnivorous than man.

Again, the teeth of the orang-outang, which is frugivorous in its habits, bear a much greater likeness to those of the flesh-eating animals than the teeth of man; so that it is evident our race is farther removed by nature from the carnivora than is the race of apes, which more nearly resembles us.

Let anyone who is still troubled with doubts on this subject examine the jaws of his dog and compare them honestly with his own. He will not find in **his** mouth the uneven, sharp-pointed incisors, or the projecting tusks of his dumb favourite; but, on the contrary, he will observe that his teeth are short, broad, and blunt, closely adjoining one another like those of the deer and kine. Thomas Bell, in a work entitled "***The Anatomy, Physiology, and Diseases of the Teeth***," remarks that the formation of the human jaw and teeth, as well as the character of all the organs and limbs of man, class him indubitably among the frugivorous animals. Such also is the opinion of Roget, Broussonet, Ray, Sir E. Home, Baron Cuvier, Linnaeus, Gassendi, Sylvester Graham, Professor Lawrence, and other eminent and learned physiologists and natural philosophers.

But, again, we have the witness of instinct on our side. We hear a vast deal about the infallible and sacred character of instinct. Theologians appeal to the natural instinct of man as a proof that he is a religious animal; and, apart from Revelation, it is on human instinct that they rely as the chief assurance of immortality. Let us inquire, then, in what direction instinct leads us with regard to our choice of food. Man under his noblest aspects is compassionate, gentle, unselfish, benign; he has a horror of injustice and of bloodshed; he abhors cruelty. If he sees any creature in pain or distress, he instantly conceives it is his duty to assist and relieve it. His spirit is moved to indignation at the sight of oppression or tyranny. He feels that war is a lamentable barbarism, and endeavours, accordingly, to settle international disputes by means of arbitration. Carnage and the odour of death occasion him the deepest repugnance. He is a peace-maker, and he believes that title constitutes his highest claim to be called a child of God.

How absurd and inconsistent to suppose that such a being as this ought to feed like a beast of prey! How ridiculous to invest him with the sanguinary desires of the tiger or the vulture! If the appetite for flesh were a true instinct in man, he would share the savage disposition of the carnivora; it would be a pleasure to him to kill and tear his victim, and the sight of blood would be an agreeable titillation to his hunger. The carnivorous tribes delight in slaughter because slaughter is normal to their nature. But civilised man, on the contrary, has so great an aversion to bloodshed and to the sight of death, that he is apt to shudder on passing a butcher's stall, to quicken his steps, and to thank Heaven that he does not belong to so repulsive a trade. He employs other people of coarser organisation than himself, men who are the helots of modern times, to slaughter victims for his use; and when, finally, their limbs are brought to his table, prepared by the art of cookery, he further disguises the taste and appearance of them with unwholesome sauces, fiery condiments, poisonous seasonings, and fantastic garnishes.

How I should like to compel all flesh-eating men and women to kill their own meat! Conceive the delicate lady of the period going out, knife in hand, to slaughter her victims for the next day's dinner! Imagine the clergyman, whose mission it is to preach mercy and benevolence, taking his pole-axe from the shelf and sallying forth to his cattle-shed intent on taking innocent life! What a vulgar picture! What a coarse and indelicate conception! Quite so! But this is just what would be natural enough if human instincts were really carnivorous. Observe the little child, – for in childhood you have the nature of man in its purest and most uncorrupted state. I lately saw a little girl weep bitterly for hours and refuse all consolation because a favourite rabbit had been killed for the mid-day meal. Let such training continue, and by and by that child will become hardened by habit, depraved by contact with a world which lives amiss, and be no longer moved by the sweet impulses of pity.

In the recent accounts of the Tichborne trial, most of us read the testimony given to the claimant's identity by a metropolitan butcher. In the course of his examination it was elicited that butchers, while employed in the slaughterhouse, are compelled to walk about upon clogs to preserve their feet from being soaked with blood. The floor of the slaughter-house is a great red pool of steaming blood! Can anything be pictured more awful, more infernal, than such a sight? Conceive what manner of men these unfortunate slaughterers must become after a few years of constant familiarity with scenes and odours of this character, in which it is also theirs to enact the chief horrible part! What chance have they, do you think, of being gentle, refined, or noble-hearted men? Can such men conceive lofty aspirations, or form high ideals? Can they appreciate pure happiness? And so long as a certain number of human souls is thus sacrificed to the debased desires of the rest of our race, must we not admit that our boasted civilisation is a chimera? Every flesh-eater is guilty, not only of shedding innocent blood at the hands of his helot, but is guilty also of causing the degradation and pollution of a human soul. The depravity and insensibility of the butcher rest upon the purchaser, who is morally responsible for retaining in a debased condition the intellect of a fellow-man.

[Here the lecturer related the incident of the butcher and the child, referred to in the first of her *Letters on Pure Diet* in **The Food Reform Magazine**.]

I confess, indeed, that I cannot perceive what logical basis for the support of the flesh-eating doctrine is left to those who affirm the wisdom of the Creator or who desire the progress of civilisation. For it follows, if the consumption of flesh be natural and necessary to man, that God must have intended his bodily appetite to do continual violence to his spiritual instincts, since he must, at the same time, have implanted in the human heart a love of gentleness and an aspiration after purity and divine benevolence, while obliging the human organisation to subsist by deeds of carnage. Such a supposition is, in the last degree, derogatory to the wisdom of God, since it maintains Him to have perpetrated a stupidity and inconsistency which the most simple of us can readily perceive. And because civilisation, with its concomitants of education, refinement, and morality, must certainly tend to increase the benignity of the human race, the opponents of Vegetarianism ought reasonably to advocate our return to a state of barbarism, that so the growing aversion to bloodshed might diminish among us, and the old ardour for battle and rapine return to the heart of mankind.

Not unfrequently, too, we are fated to hear the beautiful argument – "Animals must have been intended for the food of man; else, why were they created at all?" It really is very preposterous that man should imagine everything he beholds has been designed solely for his consumption! Are there not scores and scores of creatures which live, and move, and die around us, of which we cannot make, and have never attempted to make, any use as food? Are there not innumerable mineral and vegetable poisons throughout nature which we do not conceive ourselves in any way bound to consume? Is no creature to have a right to life for life's sake except ourselves? Nothing to exist but for our gratification? We have already observed that those creatures which men are accustomed to eat are not by any means such as God created them: man has degenerated and enfeebled them for his own ends. Obviously, therefore, the wild ox was no more created to be eaten by man than the rhinoceros or the river-horse. It would be much more logical to assert that the human races were created to be the prey of lions, bears, panthers, tigers, or wolves, which are certainly carnivorous animals, than to presume that sheep and oxen were designed to be victims for us, who are furnished with teeth and internal organs suitable for vegetable diet.

Time will not suffice me in this brief address to examine at length the objection raised against us on the head of the comparative value to the human system of mixed and of Vegetarian diet. Other writers and lecturers, vastly more fitted than I to deal with this important subject, have, already and triumphantly, vindicated our cause in this respect. Suffice it, therefore, to observe, briefly, that the origin of all nutriment is found in the vegetable kingdom; that the various articles comprised in a vegetarian dietary are more digestible than a corresponding average from the flesh of animals; that flesh-meat contains about 25 %, of nutritious matter, while rice, wheat, pease, and beans contain from 82 to 92 %, and potatoes 28 %; that one pound of bread, oatmeal, rice, or sago contains more solids than three pounds of flesh, and a pound of potatoes as much as a pound of beef. Notwithstanding this, there are persons found, usually among the ranks of ordinary medical practitioners, who may be heard to declare, with much assurance, that the principles of nutrition found in vegetables differ in character from the fibrin, albumen, and casein of animal food, and that only animal food imparts muscle and strength to the human body. But the experiments of Liebig, Dr. Lyon Playfair, Boussingault, and other distinguished chemists have established, beyond possibility of doubt, the fact that animal and vegetable substances are identical in fibrin, albumen, and casein, and that both contain precisely the same amount of azotised principle.

Moreover, vegetable diet is incontestably superior to flesh-tissue in point of purity, for the latter is often tainted or diseased in consequence of the unnatural state in which creatures bred for slaughter are habitually kept, the cramped, confined, and ill-ventilated spaces allowed them for exercise, and the unwholesome aliments on which they are fed in order to induce that abnormal deposit of fat which, though deemed a delicacy, is really a diseased condition of body. All of us are familiar enough, for example, with the sight and smell of a pig-stye. Many breeders of pigs feed their beasts upon every filthy substance that comes to hand – old sour wash, slops, the entrails of oxen and other offal. The flesh of hogs thus raised is sold for healthy pork. But even if pigs are cleanly fed and reared more expensively, it would still be better not to rear them at all. It is a very great wrong that a quantity of precious grain, which would be wholesome and nutritious as food for man, should annually be converted into poisonous hog-grease, which contains no nourishing element, and which corrupts the blood, vitiates the mind, and disorders the system of the consumer. Apart from these considerations, it is obvious that all cattle driven to market, and conveyed thither by rail or steamship, must be more or less disordered. The terror, the blows, the foul air, the fatigue, the maddening thirst these poor, animals experience during their transit, all tend to set up an abnormal and feverish condition of body; the blood becomes inflamed, the secretions disturbed, the system suffers exhaustion and irritation, and the result is febrility and diseased tissue. Indeed, nothing less could be expected.

But while on the subject of animal disorders, I

should like to draw your attention to a few significant particulars connected with it. Did you ever reflect how strange a thing it is that man, the master of creation, appears, more than any other creature, to be the prey of disease and premature death? **Wild** animals rarely suffer from disease; they die of old age, or by accident. Oxen and sheep and other domesticated beasts are more frequently disordered, but the proportion and variety of even their complaints is not to be compared to those of man. For the truth is, as I once heard a preacher say, that every creature, except man, and those unfortunate animals whom man has seduced, obeys the will of God and fulfils its nature. Man suffers disease because he has sinned. "God made him upright," says a wise writer, "but men have sought out many inventions." And it is one of Nature's most remarkable laws that the children must bear the iniquity of the fathers. Nothing is able to save a man from the transgressions of his ancestors. Ages ago, our progenitors forsook the course of diet prescribed for them by Nature, and forgot that original command of Divine wisdom, "Behold, I give you every herb which is on the face of all the earth, and every tree in which is the fruit of a tree; to you it shall be for meat." How impious to assert that the food which Divine appointment selected for man is inadequate for his sustenance, unsuited to his organisation! Yet this is the foolish and irreverent idea which man conceived, and upon which he acted. And Nature, who forgives nothing, has visited the crime upon every successive generation. The predisposition to such diseases as gout, consumption, or heart complaint, is usually an inheritance from parents or ancestors who have violated the most obvious conditions of hygiene. Nevertheless we go on, year after year, in the same vicious excesses, indulging our palates with improper food, and compelling our innocent babes to partake of the same nauseous diet, till they, too, learn to like and to crave for it. Thus our whole systems have become vitiated, easily disturbed, the prey of all manner of maladies; and recent years have added incalculably to the mischief by building up, upon this basis of flesh-diet, a culinary code of luxurious living which will, by and by, be the ruin of England, as it was in old times the ruin of the Roman Empire. All simplicity, all healthfulness, have disappeared from our mode of cooking; every viand of which we partake is disguised alike in name and appearance, and the very praise and glory of kitchen art seems to consist in making the taste and the look of any particular dish as unlike its original component elements as possible. Glancing over a fashionable cookery-book the other day, I lighted on a string of "ménus" for family dinners. I could not recognise in the catalogue of soups, meats, and puddings furnished a single English name, not could I form the least notion of the appearance or taste of a single article! Fortunes are expended in these days over the preparation of a lunch, a breakfast, or a supper, not to mention the fabulous sums lavished on civic or on royal dinners. The entertainment lately given to the Shah of Persia, at the Guildhall, is estimated to have cost forty thousand pounds. With such statistics as this before us, what can we hope for the health prospects of the rising generation? Luxury and gluttony have their record in every newspaper we take up, in every fashionable chronicle or advertisement that comes to hand. English men and women cannot meet in committee, nor assist a charity, nor join in a religious service, without supplementing the act with inordinate eating and drinking. In old times, even in the age of our grandparents, flesh-meat once a day used to be considered sufficient. But the people of our generation, in the same class of life, accustom themselves to hot meat breakfasts, and to the same diet at lunch and dinner. Thus the history of the world repeats itself, and the rebuke which Horace applied to the Romans of his time is verified of us also: "The age of our fathers hath produced us still more wicked, hereafter to leave a posterity more vicious still."

There is yet another point in connection with Vegetarianism which influences my mind very strongly. As I have not elsewhere encountered any reference to this particular consideration, it may not be amiss to record my opinion upon it here. I allude to the aspects of Vegetarian diet as they affect the subject of woman's emancipation. Conservatives in social and domestic matters are constantly urging upon us the pretended fact that one of the chief duties of woman is – to cook. And the exigencies of modern cookery have grown to such an alarming extent that, if women are to satisfy all the present demands of this luxurious age with regard to the pleasures of the table, they certainly will have no time left them for serious pursuits. Now, the Vegetarian system is pre-eminently calculated to rescue women from the drudgery which threatens them in respect of the culinary art. Simple and wholesome cooking, such as we advocate, would relieve the sex from more than half the hard toil and anxiety of the present ***régime***, while it would promote the health of every member of the household. "At least four-fifths of all the money expended for medicines and medical advice," says a writer in the **Science of Health Journal**, "are paid because of the diseases of women and children. And nine-tenths of all the care, nursing, night-watching, and privation of sleep and rest because of sick children are performed and suffered by women." Hygienic diet would get rid of almost all this vexation and expense, for over-stuffing and improper food are the fruitful causes of both adult and childish complaints. The Medical Society in New York, on one of its festive occasions, toasted woman in the following terms: "Woman, God's best gift to man, and the chief support of the doctors." The sentiment, if not poetical, is, at least, significant, and should point a sting at the conscience of every housewife who prepares or sanctions the consumption of unwholesome and luxurious diet. In these days of close competition and expensive living, what a boon would the adoption of Vegetarian habits prove to young couples with small incomes! How it would lighten the anxiety of husband and wife! Love would then become a possibility for almost every man and woman, early marriages would be feasible, and the advent of children would cease to be a cause of distress. A young lady with whom I am acquainted recently engaged herself to a struggling lieutenant with scanty means. All her friends exclaimed against the absurdity and folly of the proceeding. "How are the butcher's bills to be paid with two hundred a year," they cried, "and meat a shilling a pound?" But a Vegetarian brother of mine observed very gravely, "If only they knew **how** to live, two hundred a year would amply suffice them."

But we shall be told, perhaps, that in cold climates like our own, flesh-meat is necessary to sustain the heat of our organisation. Chemistry will inform you that vegetable diet is, at least, quite as rich in heat-forming principle as animal food, and for proof the querist may be referred to the evidence afforded by the contrasted habits of the Finns and Lapps dwelling in the same bleak latitude. The former live upon grain, the latter on flesh. And as a result the Finns are strong, vigorous, well-grown men, while the Lapps, on the contrary, are stunted and diminutive.

One of the most sturdy agitations of the day is the movement in favour of abolishing the Game Laws. It is conceived by many thoughtful persons that there must be something grievously amiss in a system which permits the expulsion of human inhabitants from large tracts of land, and the prohibition of tillage, in order to stock preserves with game and deer for the purposes of so-called sport. The people of England are beginning to assert that they have a right to their country; that it is unjust to parcel it out into private wildernesses and wastes, from which all human feet, save those of the owner and his friends, are to be excluded; that, in short, the landed system of our country needs radical reform. It is not my province to enter into the **political** bearings of this subject; but the occasion will, I think, permit me to say a few words with regard to the demoralising tendency of private sport. Week after week our newspapers record the wholesale slaughter of hares, pheasants, grouse, and other animals in the preserves of some illustrious member of the Upper House; and it is written for our learning that His Royal Highness, or his Ducal Grace, bagged, like any poulterer, so many head of game. I am not going to enlarge on the sufferings of these unlucky creatures, exposed so cruelly to the inexperienced fire of nervous or of unpractised shooters, but rather, I wish to point out the pernicious effects of such amusements upon the persons who indulge in them, and, through them, upon the moral tone of the country. At Hurlingham, where the members of the nobility accustom themselves to do butcher's work on a number of tame and defenceless pigeons, it is forbidden by the laws of sport to aim twice at the same bird. If, therefore, the shooter should not be sufficiently dexterous to kill his victim at first fire, the wretched pigeon falls wounded on the grass, and pants away its life as speedily as it may. And while bird after bird is let out of its narrow little trap to meet a death it has not much chance of escaping, creatures, with the forms and the faces of women, sit by it in their laces and ribbons, and look on with a smile – creatures who are destined to become the mothers of, at least, some of our rising aristocracy.

Then we have the battues, which are, perhaps, more horrible and un-English in detail than even the sport at Hurlingham, and these also are attended by ladies. In pastimes of such description there is no real healthy sport, but only a gratification of the savage desire to kill and shed blood, a desire unnatural to civilised man, and which, so long as it is fostered and encouraged by a luxurious and excessive system of stimulating diet, will place the persons who manifest it outside the pale of this century's philosophy, and will greatly retard the progress and enlightenment of our race. Long since, the voice of the nation condemned bear-baiting, bull-fighting, and all the kindred sports which involved barbarous and demoralising cruelty. Very lately the law inflicted its punishment on a number of persons belonging to the upper ranks of society who had been found guilty of taking part at a cock-fight. But the spirit of these deadly games still survives at Hurlingham, and in the park-preserves of many a noble peer. Will the nation have nothing more to say on the subject?

Only a few weeks ago I had a short conversation with a clever and well-informed clergyman of the English Church, who is also a classical master at one of our chief public schools. He told me that he had just been preaching a sermon at the school-chapel upon the Christian duty of kindness to animals. He gave me his sermon, in manuscript, and we commented on it together. I remarked: "As far as it goes, I think the advice you give most excellent; but in my opinion it does not reach far enough." "No," returned he, with great honesty; "I admit your logic. When I had finished my sermon I felt that, to carry my argument to its true conclusions, I ought to have recommended abstinence from flesh as food. It sounds foolish and inconsistent to warn boys of the wickedness of teasing or robbing a few wild birds and animals, while tacitly admitting the propriety of shedding the blood of any number of creatures daily in order to gratify a selfish appetite. I know I have been illogical, but everybody else is the same. It would never do to preach Vegetarianism in the pulpit: I should have my bishop down on me!"

Alas! alas! Here, then, we have the very pith and core of our difficulty with the people! Vegetarianism is supposed to be at variance with the dictates of religion! Now, on this point I am prepared to deny resolutely the possibility of finding in the Jewish Scriptures a single phrase condemnatory of vegetable diet, given with the authority of Divine command. There are, on the contrary, many passages which plainly indicate the displeasure with which the God of Israel regarded the adoption of carnivorous habits by man. So many persons have instanced the original ordinance delivered to Adam with regard to his diet, that I think it superfluous to dwell on the subject here. For the same reason, I pass over the record of the punishment incurred by the early Jews, in the desert at Sinai, in consequence of their lust after the flesh-pots of Egypt; and, in respect of this incident, I will merely remark that the wandering Israelites could not possibly have been accustomed to feed on the flocks and herds which accompanied them, else the demand for flesh would have been beyond measure absurd and superfluous. It is evident that the vegetable manna described as "angel's food" was their only aliment until the supply of quails arrived in the camp. But these details have been, one and all, so ably handled, that I prefer to take other ground. Nevertheless, in order that no one may have reason to accuse me of unfairness in dealing with this part of my subject, I will, while on the treatment of texts, instance and examine the only passage in the whole Bible which appears unfavourable to the tenets of Vegetarianism. It occurs in the First Epistle of St Paul to Timothy: "Now the Spirit speaketh expressly, that in the latter times some shall depart from the faith, giving heed to spirits of error, (...) forbidding to marry, and commanding to abstain from meats, which God hath created to be received with thanksgiving; for every creature of God is good, and nothing to be rejected, for it is sanctified by the word of God and prayer." Now, in the first place, I observe that these Epistles of St Paul, and of other early Christian writers, although they have received the sanction of the Church, are not to be regarded as the direct communications of the Divine Being, nor to be invested with any superstitious awe. They are simply the utterances of minds which reflected all the early errors and prejudices of the infant Christian community. If we want proof of this, we need not seek far. The Epistles are full of exhortations, and warnings of the speedy dissolution of the world, plainly showing that their writers, one and all, laboured under the delusion that they were, even then, living in the last days. How far they erred in this respect we all know. Again: it happens that this special passage about abstaining from meat was written against an ancient sect of heretics, called the Manicheans, which had just then arisen to vex the orthodox. These Manicheans held that all **flesh** was from an evil principle, and of the devil's creation. Hence St Paul, who, by the way, erroneously imagined the appearance of this sect to prognosticate the arrival of the last day, assures the faithful that flesh is by no means the result of an evil principle, but quite otherwise, the work of God Himself. This fact no modern Vegetarian denies; but, so far to the contrary, **because** every living being is the work of God, he abhors the idea of defacing its beauty, shedding its innocent blood, and robbing it of the life he cannot give. Observe, too, that the progress of mankind and the advance of human intellect have caused many of the precepts contained in the Epistles to be set aside, with the full consent of the greatest intellects among us. St Paul has laid down several maxims with regard to the mutual behaviour of masters and slaves, for the word rendered "servant" in our English text is really "slave." And, for a long time, one of the arguments against the abolition of negro slavery was founded on the Biblical passage – "Cursed is Canaan; a servant of servants shall he be." Slavery also was practised under priestly sanction among the chosen race, as the Pentateuch clearly shows. Yet we have abolished the buying and selling of human beings with the hearty consent and approval of modern Christendom. And, in like manner, the Apostolic injunctions with regard to the position and treatment of woman are receiving their dismissal from the civilised code of morality. St Paul strongly deprecated any attempt to bestow liberty upon womankind. Later on, the Christians brutally murdered a pagan lady, named Hypatia, who offended their sense of the proprieties by lecturing in public. So, you see, that if the doctrines of St Paul with regard to feminine conduct obtained today, as they once did, I should not certainly be permitted to address you, with impunity, from this platform. And, once more: although St Paul made use of the language I have quoted with regard to the eating of meat, it is, nevertheless, clear that all the chief saints of the religion he advocated were strict Vegetarians in diet. St John the Baptist was a notable example of Vegetarianism; the locust-plant of the East and the honey of the wild bee supplying all his needs. And after St Paul, or almost contemporary with him, lived St Matthew the Evangelist, Augustine, John Chrysostom, Antony, Hilarion, Martin of Tours, Ambrose of Milan, Benedict, Francis Xavier, Catherine of Sienna, Dominic, Theresa, Bernard the Great, Gregory, Aphratus, Serapion, Genevieve, Columba, Charles Borromeo, Philip Neri, Alphonsus, Ignatius, all of them rigid abstainers from flesh, besides an army of hermits, Fathers of the Desert, and principals of ecclesiastical orders. And, in more modern times, we count among the ranks of Vegetarians such men as Byron, Shelley, Wordsworth, Sir Isaac Newton, Sir Richard Phillips, Dr. Lambe, Ritson, Haller, Howard, Swedenborg, and the reformer Wesley; while among the wise thinkers and teachers of heathen times, Pythagoras, the philosopher, was eminent in condemning the use of flesh as food, and his practice and opinions were also those of Zeno, Diogenes, Plato, Plutarch, Produs, Apollonius of Tyana, a seer and a worker of miracles; Porphyry, Plautus, and many others.

Surely we cannot suppose that all these Christian saints and famous philosophers erred throughout their lives; or that a solitary expression of apostolic opinion in one Epistle is to be taken as outweighing and condemning the belief and practice of so many good and wise persons; to say nothing of the **direct** contradiction which the passage in question offers to many other texts throughout the Scriptures of much higher and Diviner authority.

I shall, therefore, beg you to reflect that, although it is right to regard sacred writings with every reverence, they ought not, by any means, to be understood as containing **all** that God has to say to the world and to our souls. God has not ceased to exist, nor is His voice silenced. As in old times He spoke to our race by the lips of men of poetic or prophetic genius, so also He yet speaks in the wonderful language of Science. Every truth which comes to light is God's truth, and to nothing but error can it be dangerous. Little by little, as the world is able to bear it, God uncovers the splendour of His divine face. Every new discovery in anatomy, physiology, chemistry, geology, or any other branch of learning, is a word of God, as truly and as powerfully as though it were the utterance of a Daniel or of a St John. "I have many things to say unto you," quoth the Messiah, "but ye cannot bear them now. But when the Spirit of Truth cometh, He shall lead you into all truth." Yes, the world must be **led** towards the light, step after step, and by slow degrees. Does not the very word "**lead**" convey to our apprehension the sense of **gradual** approach? Therefore, to those wise and philosophic minds who stand before their brothers in the great army of advancing humanity, does the Divine Mind reveal, continually, more and more of itself; inspiring them with the burning desire to enlighten others, and, so doing, to rise into still closer union with the pure spirituality they covet. For the God of the Holy Scriptures is also the God of Nature; and, since it is impossible for God to contradict Himself, these two must agree, and must be equally divine. Whatever, therefore, we find to be the teaching of science, we must accept with perfect and entire reverence as being the true Word of God. Science is the Apocalypse of To-Day, the revelation vouchsafed to the present age. Not alone in the leaves of a printed volume, the text of which has undergone many vicissitudes and translations, many losses, additions, and interpolations, and the intentions of which often lie hid in obscure orientalisms, parables, and enigmas – not alone in the pages of our Jewish and Christian Scriptures, does the Voice of God address us, but far more clearly, majestically, and forcibly in the living Nature around us. His Word is written on star, and plant, and stone. He speaks to us in the thousand voices of the earth, bidding us aspire ever upward towards the perfect day; bidding us rise through sphere after sphere, hating and casting from our ascending spirits the garment spotted by the flesh. He bids us abstain from the pollution of blood, and revert to the original purity in which we were created, for thus only can we hope again to make our world a Paradise. Then the dream of Isaiah will be realised, and the Kingdom of God shall come in its fulness: "The wolf shall dwell with the kid, and the leopard shall lie down with the lamb; and the calf, and the lion, and the sheep shall abide together, and a little child shall lead them. They shall not hurt, nor shall they kill in all my holy mountain, for the earth shall be filled with the knowledge of the Lord, as the covering waters of the sea."

Vainly, to-day, we dream of universal peace — vainly we talk about abolishing war among nations, while we are still content to live like brutes of prey. As long as men feed like tigers, they will retain the tiger's nature. Universal peace will be impossible until man abjures the diet of blood. Thus, I regard Vegetarianism as the ultimate and the only means of the world's redemption. Even the commonest and most popular conception of the condition of things which will obtain under the immediate reign of Christ precludes the anticipation of bloodshed. Then, as Isaiah says in another of his prophecies, "He that killeth an ox shall be, in the sight of the Lord, as if he slew a man."

Therefore, let us rid ourselves as soon as we may of the absurd fancy that science and the instincts of humanity are less holy or less venerable than the text of Scripture. We shall yet see the day when no imaginary distinction will be drawn between so-called **sacred** and so-called **secular** knowledge. All knowledge is equally sacred. Nature can unfold nothing to us but God. Whatever theory, whatever aspiration receives the sanction of science, and the approval of virtue, is, undoubtedly, the inspiration of the Father of Spirits, demanding our ready and perfect obedience to its dictates. And I know that at some distant day, now, indeed, perhaps very remote, the message we preach in a corner will become the religion of great nations. To us, meanwhile, it belongs to inaugurate the Golden Age with words of entreaty and appeal, whose spirit and whose burden shall be these:

> *Rise, human soul!* "*Arise*
>   *and fly*
> *The reeling Faun, the sensual*
>   *feast;*
> *Move upward, working out*
>   *the beast,*
> *And let the wolf and tiger*
>   *die!*"

---

1. A lecture given by Anna Kingsford, reprinted from ***The Ideal in Diet: Selections from the Writings of Anna Bonus Kingsford***.

8. FROM ADDRESSES TO VEGETARIANS

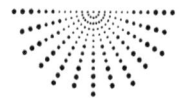

I[1] ALWAYS speak with the greatest delight and satisfaction in the presence of my friends the members of the Vegetarian Society. With them I am quite at my ease, I have no reservation, I have no dissatisfaction. This is not the case when I speak for my friends the Anti-Vivisectionists, the Anti-Vaccinationists, the Spiritualists, or the advocates of freedom for women. I always feel that such of these as are not abstainers from flesh-food have unstable ground under their feet, and it is my great regret that, when helping them in their good works, I cannot openly and publicly maintain what I so ardently believe – that the Vegetarian movement is the bottom and basis of all other movements towards Purity, Freedom, Justice, and Happiness.

I think it was Benjamin D'Israeli who said that

we had stopped short at Comfort, and had mistaken it for Civilisation, content to increase the former at the expense of the latter. Not a day passes without the perspicacity of this remark coming forcibly before me. Comfort, luxury, indulgence, and ease abound in this age, and in this part of the world; but, alas! of Civilisation we have as yet acquired but the veriest rudiments. Civilisation means not mere physical ease, but moral and spiritual Freedom – Sweetness and Light – with which the customs of the age are in most respects at dire enmity. I named just now freedom for women. One of the greatest hindrances to the advancement and enfranchisement of the sex is due to the luxury of the age, which demands so much time, study, money, and thought to be devoted to what is called the "pleasures of the table." A large class of men seems to believe that women were created chiefly to be "housekeepers," a term which they apply almost exclusively to ordering dinners and superintending their preparation. Were this office connected only with the garden, the field, and the orchard, the occupation might be truly said to be refined, refining, and worthy of the best and most gentle lady in the land. But, connected as it is actually with slaughter-houses, butchers' shops, and dead carcases, it is an occupation at once unwomanly, inhuman, and barbarous in the extreme. Mr. Ruskin has said that the criterion of a beautiful action or of a noble thought is to be found in song, and that an action about which we cannot make a poem is not fit for humanity. Did he ever apply this test to flesh-eating? [2] Many a lovely poem, many a beautiful picture, may be made about gardens and fruit-gathering, and the bringing home of the golden produce of harvest, or the burden of the vineyards, with groups of happy boys and girls, and placid, mild-eyed oxen bending their necks under their fragrant load. But I defy anyone to make beautiful verse or to paint beautiful pictures about slaughter-houses, running with streams of steaming blood, and terrified, struggling animals felled to the ground with pole-axes; or of a butcher's stall hung round with rows of gory corpses, and folks in the midst of them bargaining with the ogre who keeps the place for legs and shoulders and thighs and heads of the murdered creatures! What horrible surroundings are these for gentle and beautiful ladies! The word "wife" means, in the old Saxon tongue, a "weaver," and that of "husband" means, of course, a "husbandman." "Lady," too, is a word originally signifying "loaf-giver." In these old words have come down to us a glimpse of a fair picture of past times. The wife, or weaver, is the spinner, the maker, whose function it is to create forms of beauty and decorative art, to brighten, adorn, and make life lovely. Or if, as "lady" of the house, we look on her in the light of the provider and dispenser of good things, it is not loathsome flesh of beasts that she gives, but bread – sweet and pure, and innocent type of all human food. As for the man, he is the cultivator of the ground, a sower of grain, a tiller of the field. I would like to see these old times back, with all their sweet and tender Arcadian homeliness, in the place of the ugly lives which most folks lead in our modern towns, whose streets are hideous, above all at night, with their crowded gin-palaces, blood-smeared butchers' stalls, reeling drunkards, and fighting women. People talk to me sometimes about peace conventions, and ask me to join societies for putting down war. I always say: "You are beginning at the wrong end, and putting the cart before the horse." If you want people to leave off fighting like beasts of prey, you must first get them to leave off living like beasts of prey. You cannot reform institutions without first reforming men. Teach men to live as human beings ought to live, to think wisely, purely, and beautifully, and to have noble ideas of the purpose and meaning of Humanity, and they will themselves reform their institutions. Any other mode of proceeding will result only in a patchwork on a worthless fabric, a whitening of a sepulchre full of dead men's bones and all uncleanness. Flesh-meats and intoxicating drinks – the pabulum of Luxury – are the baneful coil of hydra-headed Vice, whose ever-renewing heads we vainly strike, while leaving the body of the dragon still untouched. Strike there – at the heart – at the vitals of the destructive monster, and the work of Heracles, the Redeemer, is accomplished.

∼

I have stood so often on this and on other platforms throughout England, as well as in Scotland and Switzerland, to speak to my friends about the physiological, chemical, anatomical, and economical aspects of the non-flesh diet, that to-night, for a change, I am going to take another and a higher line. We will, therefore, if you please, take "as read" all the vindications of our mode of living furnished by various scientific arguments: that we have the organisation of the fruit-eater; that the constituent elements of vegetable food furnish all the necessary force and material of bodily vigour; that it is cheaper to buy beans and meal than to buy pork and suet; that land goes further and supports more people under a vegetable cultivation than when laid out for pasture, and so forth. All these arguments, more or less eloquently and clearly formulated, most of you have by heart, and those who have not may buy them all for sixpence of the Vegetarian Society. So I am going to talk to you to-night about quite another branch of our subject, the loftiest and fruitfulest branch of the whole tree. I am going to tell you that I see in the doctrine we are here to preach the very culmination and crown of the Gentle Life, that Life which, in some way, we all of us in our best moments long to live, but which it is only given now and again to some great and noble soul, almost divine, fully to realise and glorify in the eyes of the world. I said just now that "in our best moments" we all long to lead the Ideal Life. Some of us have many "best moments," and long ones too: moments that dominate and top our work-a-day efforts always, like a light of stars overhead, through which the Heaven looks down on us. Some of us, again, have very few "best moments," short and feeble, like lights over a marsh, never steadfast, always flickering in and out, and paling and flitting when we get abreast of them. With this class of persons the Ideal is very faint and unstable, while with the former it is strong and masterful. Societies like ours are made to encourage the "best moments" of the weakly, and to glorify those of the strong. Societies like ours are made to train soldiers and provide them with leaders to fight for the Ideal. Beginners and feeble folk cannot stand without encouragement in the teeth of a hot fire, nor rush upon the enemy unless some hero heads them and shows the way. The Ideal Life, the Gentle Life, has many enemies, and the weapons used by these are various. They are pseudo-scientific, pseudo-religious, pseudo-philanthropic, pseudo-aesthetic, and pseudo-utilitarian. And the enemies are of all ranks, professions, and interests.

But of all the weapons used, the most deadly, the most terrific, is – Ridicule. Yes, Ridicule slays its tens of thousands! To be laughed at is far more awful to average mortals than to be preached at, groaned at, cursed at. It is the weapon which the journalists almost always handle with the greatest facility. These are the men who laugh for their living. They have replaced, in modern days, the paid domestic jesters of olden times. Every town keeps its paid jester now in the office of its local paper, just as, a few centuries back, great nobles kept their man in cap and motley to crack jokes on the guests at table. We have not changed in manners, but in manner only. And the very first thing that Reformers have to do is to get over minding the man in motley. Let him laugh. He cannot argue. Laughing is his stock-in-trade. If he laugh not too coarsely, and avoid blaspheming, he is, after all, very harmless. It is his privilege to laugh at all that is new and unwonted. All children do that, and the man in motley is but a clever child. Why let him knock you down with his fool's truncheon? Wince, and shrink, and expostulate: he sees his advantage then, and belabours you pitilessly. But heed him not, and go on doing your work with a great heart as though it were a royal thing to do, and he will soon be off to some other quarry. Only be sure in your own mind that you are **right**; only be set in dead earnest on keeping that royal thing in clear view and working up to it, and the Ideal will reward you by becoming the Real and Actual. It is not necessary to go very far afield to find this royal work. It does not lie – for most of us – in setting out to accomplish some vast task. Most of us will find it in just simply and calmly shaping out and lifting up our own lives so as to beautify and perfect and unify them, being just and merciful to all men and all creatures. We Vegetarians carry the Ideal a stage lower, and, therefore, a stage higher than do other folk. We find the duty to the lowliest the duty completest in blessing.

Let me tell you a story. Once, in the far-away old days of romance, there was a Christian Knight of peerless repute, whose greatest longing and dearest hope it was to have the Vision of the Holy Grail. The Holy Grail is the name given in chivalry to the Chalice of the Altar containing the Sacred Blood of Christ, and this was said to be shown in a Vision by God to those whom He judged worthy of the sight of this supreme symbol of His Grace, in the moment when they pleased Him most. Well, the Knight of whom I speak, in pursuance of the Object of his desire, joined the Crusaders, and performed prodigies of valour and wonderful feats of arms in battle against the Infidels, but all in vain; he had no Vision and remained unblessed. Then he left Palestine and went and laid aside his sword in a monastery, and lived a life of long penance and meditation, desiring always a sight of the Holy

Grail. But that, too, was in vain. At last, sorrowful and almost despairing, he returned homeward to his domain. As he drew near his castle, he saw gathered about its gates a crowd of beggars, sick, maimed, aged and infirm, old men, women, babes, and children – all who were left behind on the land while the hale and hearty went to fight the Saracens. Then he said to his squire: "What are these?" "They are beggars." the squire answered, "who can neither work nor fight. They clamour for bread; but why heed such a herd of useless, despicable wretches? Let me drive them away." "Nay," said the Knight, touched to the heart, "I have slain many abroad, let me save some at home. Call these poor folk together, give them bread and drink; let them be wanned and clothed." And lo! as the words passed his lips, a light from heaven fell upon him, and, looking up, he saw, at last, the longed-for Vision of the Holy Grail! Yes, that humble, simple, homely duty of charity was more precious in the Eyes Divine than all his deeds of prowess in the field of arms, or his long devotions in the cloister!

And so with us. Who so poor, so oppressed, so helpless, so mute and uncared for, as the dumb creatures who serve us – they who, but for us, must starve, and who have no friend on earth if man be their enemy? Even these are not too low for pity, nor too base for justice. And, without fear of irreverence or slight on the holy name that

Christians love, we may truly say of them, as of the captive, the sick, and the hungry: "Inasmuch as ye do it unto the least of these, my brethren, ye do it unto me."

For, as St Francis of Assisi has told us, all the creatures of God's hand are brethren. "My sisters the birds," he was wont to say – "My brothers the kine in the meadows." The essential of true justice is the sense of solidarity. All creatures, from highest to lowest, stand hand in hand before God. Nor shall we ever begin to spiritualise our lives and thoughts, to lighten and lift ourselves higher, until we recognise this solidarity, until we learn to look upon the creatures of God's hand, not as mere subjects for hunting and butchery, for dissecting and experimentation, but as ***living souls*** with whom, as well as with the sons of men, God's covenant is made.

---

1. Two examples of addresses given by Anna Kingsford to the Vegetarian Society (from ***The Life of Anna Kingsford***, *vol.* ii. pp. 223-227).
2. Edward Maitland says: "So, after all, Mr. Ruskin is 'no vegetarian'; but, like his fellow-prophet of Chelsea [Carlyle], his principles are one thing, his practice another. (...) He can write exquisitely of beauty, honour, tenderness, 'fields and sunshine, babes and all that sort of thing,' and all the while be a patron of shambles, with their inevitable moral ugliness of long-drawn distress and barbarous violent death to gentle-eyed herbivores, and degradation unspeakable to a vast class of fellow-men.

And this, too, when Science has demonstrated that man is, by his structure, adapted to be an eater only of grains and fruits; when Common Sense assures us that Nature must know best what is good for us; and when History shows that all great reformers, not of institutions merely, but of men themselves – the Pythagorases, the Buddhas, and Sages and Saints innumerable – have made it the first step towards the perfection preached by Mr. Ruskin, that their disciples should so order their mode of sustaining themselves as to involve no shock to the moral sentiments."

9. EVOLUTION AND FLESH-EATING

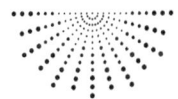

I[1] HOLD that Darwin's theory of development is right in principle, even though it may be a little inaccurate in detail; and I am therefore prepared to admit ***a priori***, in accord with his views and with the inspired declaration of Genesis, that "creation" has been, and still is, a process of evolution, proceeding from a lower to a higher grade.

Man, then, having developed from the Ape-Men (of Haeckel), and those Ape-Men being themselves the product of a lower type, all having, as have the Simian tribes to-day, the teeth and alimentary canal of frugivorous creatures, it is clear that Man became Man by means of fruit-eating. He did not, and could not develop out of the Carnivora. Humanity, therefore, is the product, not of flesh-eating, but of fruit-eating; and it is certain from history and from internal evidence that the "Golden Age," which was distinguished by the familiar intercourse of Man with God, or with "the gods," was an age of innocence and of abstinence from blood. Therefore, the more our mode of life removes us from the possibility of the privileges and spiritual powers which Man then enjoyed, the more it tends to degrade us; and the more, on the other hand, our diet accords with that of the Golden Age, the more it tends to develop our faculties and to **redeem** us. For there has been a Fall, and that Fall has lost to us, for the time being, the Perfect Humanity (the subject is a vast one, and I can only indicate its bearings here).

You must not overlook the fact that not all the races of Man have become habitual eaters of flesh. There are whole nations and tribes, especially in the East, who have adhered, and who still adhere, by religious tradition to fruit and herb-eating, and the structure of their internal organs differs in no way from that of the European flesh-eating nations. But there is in this question of "adaptation" an element which I venture to suspect you equally overlook. A man's physical organism is made by his Spirit, and the spirits of many men are of such a nature and of such a pedigree that they oblige the body they control to nourish itself upon grosser particles than are necessary to the sustenance of bodies inhabited and controlled by higher and more advanced spirits.

Perhaps I fail to make my meaning clear to you, for it is probable the idea may be a wholly new one to you. Observation of individuals, however, will convince you that I am right. In fact, a particular system of diet is not hereditary in many cases, and we often hear it affirmed with truth, "What suits one does not suit another"; or, in more homely phrase, "One man's meat is another man's poison." We adapt ourselves to our food – it is not our food which is adapted to us. If the inner and true Man be pure, his dietary will necessarily befit him, for he will be unable to assimilate gross and carnivorous modes of life to the purposes of and the nourishment of his finer organism. If a man should tell me that he has convinced himself by trial that his "internal organs are adapted only for a mixed diet," I should not wish to contradict him, but he would be wholly unable to convince Me that *my* organs are in a similar condition. It is my belief that there are among men as many different species, races, types, and orders as there are among the various kinds of animals. One man is a lion or a fox, while another is a dove or a gazelle. In this respect, one may cite Plato in the **Phaedrus**, when he says: "Rather do I inquire about myself, whether I happen to be a beast with more folds and more furious than Typhon, or whether I am not a gentler and more simple animal naturally partaking of a modest and divine condition."

You will gather, madam, from what I have

written that your question appears to me to involve other considerations than a merely material mode of looking at Humanity. But, as regards the simply material view, you may rest assured that there exists nothing in the anatomical structure of Man to warrant the supposition that he has become transformed into a carnivorous animal, seeing how distinctly comparative anatomy declares to the contrary.

---

1. From a letter written by A.K. to Miss C–.

Copyright © 2021 by ALICIA EDITIONS
All rights reserved.
Credits: CANVA.COM
No part of this book may be reproduced in any form or by any electronic or mechanical means, including information storage and retrieval systems, without written permission from the author, except for the use of brief quotations in a book review.

www.ingramcontent.com/pod-product-compliance
Ingram Content Group UK Ltd.
Pitfield, Milton Keynes, MK11 3LW, UK
UKHW020708050526
12270UKWH00042B/1111